BE FIT
THROUGH
YOUR FORTIES

BE FIT THROUGH YOUR FORTIES

Eric Taylor

JAVELIN BOOKS
POOLE·NEW YORK·SYDNEY

First published in the UK 1987 by Javelin Books,
Link House, West Street, Poole, Dorset BH15 1LL

Distributed in the United States by
Sterling Publishing Co., Inc.,
2 Park Avenue, New York, NY10016

Distributed in Australia by
Capricorn Link (Australia) Pty Ltd,
PO Box 665, Lane Cove, NSW 2066

British Library Cataloguing in Publication Data

Taylor, Eric
  Be fit through your forties
  1. Physical fitness
  I. Title
  613.7   RA781

ISBN 0 7137 1844 7

Typeset by Word Perfect 99 Ltd, Bournemouth, Dorset

Printed in Great Britain by the Guernsey Press Co, Guernsey, C.I.

CONTENTS

Introduction		6
1	*You can do it!*	7
2	*Vital energy*	12
3	*Get the lean look*	21
4	*Flatten that tum!*	32
5	*Enjoy your exercise*	39
6	*Variety is the spice of life — with exercise*	44
7	*Short circuit to fitness*	51
8	*Sexual fitness*	56
9	*How to replace stress with serenity*	62
10	*Are you taking a calculated risk?*	70
11	*The secret of self-renewal*	76
12	*Take a break*	82
13	*Quickly fit after surgery*	89
14	*Why join the coronary club?*	93
15	*Avoiding cancer*	99
16	*Stop smoking*	104
17	*How about a drink?*	110
18	*Back chat*	115
19	*It's your choice*	123
Appendix I	Circuit Training Schedules	128
Appendix II	Seven-day Slimming Menus	133
Appendix III	The Fibre Chart	140
Appendix IV	Pressure Levels at Work	141
Appendix V	Ideal Weight Chart	142
Index		143

INTRODUCTION

Would you like the opportunity to look 10 or 15 years younger? Of course you would. So would most people. And it would not be for frivolous or vain reasons either. If you look younger than your age, says the American National Institute for Ageing, the chances are, your internal organs are ageing more slowly. The way you look, the way you feel, and the way you act are inseparably linked. One affects the other. Catch a glimpse of a tired, drab face in the mirror and you begin to feel and act in that way. You can lose confidence, lose interest in life and look older than you need.

You can restore the appearance of youth to the ageing face and figure, without surgery, without impossible fitness programmes, and without boringly dull diets. All those crash diets and fad fitness programmes have had their fanfares of publicity. And they have had their day. Now women, and men, want more than exciting promises. They want results, and they are not prepared to settle for anything less. Why should they?

Here, in this book, is a comprehensive programme that will fulfil the promise. It will stem the tide of ageing. The main purpose of the book is exactly that, for it brings together, in easily readable form, the latest medically approved ways in which you can help yourself to stay young longer. It can be done. It is being done. Now you can do it.

1 YOU CAN DO IT

The promise of being able to remain 40 for 20 years is surely no pipe dream. To a great extent it is in your power to make this miracle come true.

Dr Walter Noder, M.D.,
Specialist in Internal Medicine,
Rhein Lahr Clinic, West Germany.

At 40 years old you are entering the most exciting, enjoyable and satisfying years of your life! Whilst many of the pleasures of youth are still available, the rewards of maturity begin to come in. You are as close as you ever can be to enjoying the best of both worlds and you are about to discover the truth in the saying that 'Life beings at 40!' You are entering your prime and, indeed, you can stay there for much longer. *It is in your power.*

It does not take a miracle. We all know people who seem to stay younger longer than others. They remain young, physically, psychologically and sexually for 10 or 20 years after turning 39. So could we all.

The secret lies in using your own body-power to slow down the ageing process. It means changing your life style to make full use of this sophisticated force that lies within each one of us – a dynamic force that can keep us young longer, fit and healthy. It has the power to repair and regenerate body systems, protect us from the pressures of modern living, and allow us to adapt comfortably to ever changing situations. We have seen recently, for example, how many public figures have passed the 50 year mark yet still look chic and youthfully attractive. Indeed, bright-eyed Sophia Loren declares that, 'a woman gets more attractive and self-assured as she gets older.' Joan Collins, in her 50s makes the centre spread pin-up of 'Playboy' magazine, and we can see that the impish charm of a 20-year-old Shirley MacLaine is still there 30 years later. Brigitte Bardot has changed but little. Singer Petula Clark gets livelier every year and the charismatic black singer, Lena Horne, at a flourishing 67 years old, opened a new show in

London, looking delighted with life, saying, 'I sing rather better than I did 20 years ago.'

What do they have that keeps them young? It is the same dynamic body-power that we all have but they can make more use of it. Look at Hollywood's most loved leading man, Cary Grant, of whom his colleagues wrote: 'The fact that he was getting on for 70 seemed utterly unimportant both to him and to the women he took up with. If anything, he was better looking than when he was younger, his appearance astonishingly unmarked by signs of age.'

There are examples galore of celebrities who carry on regardless of age. The warm and well-loved heroine of the 1930s, Claudette Colbert, starred 50 years later in a new London Show. Concert pianist Artur Rubenstein gave his last public concert at 95 and that remarkable travel writer, Freya Stark, was on horseback in the Himalayas at 88! Pensioners all, in the old sense of the word, but proving the point that there is a power that we can harness to keep us youthfully fit and active. Yes, time is stretching for those who really want to stay young. It can for you, who are, on average, 30 years younger than these celebrities. How is it done?

First, we have to reject traditional notions of age, clear our minds of outdated ideas about declining physical ability. Remember that we are as old as our arteries, as old as we feel, as old as we look. No older!

Secondly, we must think positively about providing the right conditions for our subtle body mechanisms to work effectively in keeping us physically and mentally efficient. It is difficult for physiologists to explain how this potent force works, but we can see it acting in a number of specific examples. If you break a bone then self-healing agencies repair the fracture. Cut yourself and blood will clot of its own accord; ineffective organisms are attacked by white blood cells. The body has an amazing capacity to adjust to a wide range of conditions – it can keep your internal temperature normal whether you be in the middle of the sun-scorched Sahara or frozen Arctic. If you faint, you automatically fall flat to give your brain a better blood supply. Get something in your eye and tears will wash it out. Something lodges in your throat and you cough without thinking. Eat bad food and you will vomit and have diarrhoea to expel the poison. The whole body will respond to a frightening situation with a state of readiness; eyes dilate, muscles tense, adrenal glands stimulate all the body systems for a fight or flight. What a wonderful power we have

8

working for us. All the time. 'In at least 90 per cent of illnesses,' write
Dr Vernon Coleman, 'we are able to recover without any form of
medical treatment.'

We can use this power to keep us young longer — as we shall see in
the chapters that follow. Staying young is no longer a matter of vanity.
It is sound commonsense. We live in a most competitive world where
a high premium is put on youth. Success in a career frequently comes
from appearing young physically and mentally. Employers are
reluctant to take on men and women who look old before their time.
They look for staff with a dynamic approach to life. Job discrimination
against the over 40s is increasing even though the peak of creative
productivity remains high well into later life. Consequently it is
understandable that some men and women in their 39th year can begin
to fear ageing, with diminishing job prospects as well as the possible
loss of desirability and romance.

Fear not! It is not age that counts but the way you look and what you
can do. And this applies particularly to love and romance. Experience
in life and literature all point to the idea that chronological age matters
little. When the celebrated French singer and dancer, Mistinguette
was interviewed by a journalist towards the end of her life she was
asked whether a woman's sexual appetite diminished with age and she
replied, 'How should I know? I'm only 70.'

Years don't count: attitudes are changing. Men no longer care in the
same way what a woman's age is but what *she* is and what *she* looks
like. The same goes for women's attitude to men. Autumn and Spring
can go together. Especially when it is a young looking autumn. A well
known example is that of Charlie Chaplin. He was 54 when he
married 18-year-old Oona O'Neill. She gave him eight children and
said that the marriage was a success, 'because of the difference in age.'
When partners are well suited such a marriage has a firm foundation
for future growth. The partners grow within the marriage.

Naturally there are certain changes that come with advancing years.
We know what to expect: skin loses its elasticity which leads to
wrinkles, blood vessels harden, raising blood pressure, cartilage wears
thin so that joints become stiff and painful. But these are changes that
come not with the years we have lived but from the way we have lived.
We can change the way that we live to delay the ageing process. We do
not need 'youth drugs' or rejuvenators based on fantasy rather than
fact. Quite simply what we need to do is to reduce the needless wear

and tear of daily life and give our own body-power the right conditions for working for us.

Doctors sometimes explain the point by comparing the human body to a car. It shows signs of ageing according to the way that it is looked after. Neglect, abuse and rough handling will age it rapidly. If we look after the mechanism of the car − or the body − it will run smoothly for many more years. And, fortunately, like the car, the human body can be restored to its former glory with a thorough overhaul and service. In medical terminology: a rehabilitation programme.

This is what the separate chapters of this book will give to you. Have faith: faith in yourself, and in that miraculous body-power that we all have. No trendy fads but down-to-earth faith. Your body can cope with all kinds of setbacks and recover. You can lose more than half your lung, liver or kidney tissue without noticing any remarkable loss of function. You have heart muscles in reserve too and it often happens that people lose yards of intestine without any noticeable effect upon enjoyment of food, or digestion of it.

Have faith. It is never too late to start a rehabilitation programme. You can look younger longer, act younger, feel younger. But this is only half the story. There is a much more persuasive reason for prolonging a state of youthful fitness. That of simple survival.

Stay fit and you stay alive

An alarming number of men and women are struck down in their prime today and it is not just the middle-aged who are at risk. Heart attacks among people under 40 years old are surprisingly numerous. One adult in three in the Western World has a major or minor heart ailment. Britain is top of the league with the highest incidence of heart attacks in the world.

Women are less vulnerable until their middle 40s − or whenever the change of life occurs − but then they begin to lose their immunity to killing diseases. In the age group between 25 and 44, twice as many men as women die. Statistics are often quoted: there is little to be gained from creating fear and anxiety by emphasising them, but it is only sensible to face the hazards and avoid them.

All we need to do is to strike the right balance between all the factors affecting health and fitness; balance between activity and rest, between work and recreation, between essential nutrients and tasty treats.

There's nothing wrong in grilling a juicy steak with tasty fat running between its red muscle fibres, once in a while. But don't think that you can get away with it all the time simply because you jog three times a week. No matter how much exercise you take you still have to strike the right balance between all the other factors which affect ageing. Jim Fixx, the 'High Priest of Jogging' proved that point. In his worldwide best seller, *The Complete Book of Running* he frequently proclaimed a belief that you could eat what you liked, including foods full of cholesterol, provided you took enough exercise. In an interview with the London 'Times' he said, 'If you run you can participate fully in the ways of our civilization and get away with it.' He was wrong. He dropped dead on a jog, alone and unseen, in running shoes and shorts and was found later by a passing motorcyclist. An autopsy revealed two of his coronary arteries blocked with fatty deposits and a third half clogged.

Dramatically, Jim Fixx proved the findings of medical research that no matter how much aerobic activity you pack into your day's programme it cannot in itself counter the ageing effect of all the other factors of life which make people old before their time.

It is with this basic principle in mind that this book is written. It presents a complete programme embracing all aspects of life that affect physical and mental wellbeing. It is not just another 'Workout' book but a programme of realistic, non-trendy, rejuvenating routines which will help the body's own power to keep you fit in every way. Fit to enjoy the best years of your life. Fit to stay 39 longer. It is in your power. Now your first task is to take a close look at the fuel that provides the power. The vital energy.

2 VITAL ENERGY

In the hectic showbiz world of Broadway and London's West-End, where sparkling vitality is at a premium, the stars need a limitless source of raw, fresh energy. Where do they get it from? What do they eat?

'It's taken me years to learn about healthy eating,' said Stephanie Lawrence, the attractive singing and dancing star of the award winning show, *Evita*. 'I need food that gives me bags of energy. Enough to cope with the heavy demands of work and still have some vitality to spare.' You only have to look at this dynamic young lady whirling around the stage, and at others like her, to realise the tremendous amount of effort that goes into a performance. Abundant energy has to be readily available from easily digestible foods to keep the stars in peak condition, full of that marvellous zest for life.

It is a zest we should all like to have – and we can. But we should have to follow their example – and millions of others already doing so in the United States and Britain. They have rejected the old fashioned western diet – high in fat and sugar – and taken to the new style which provides plenty of boundless energy. But not only that. They are likely to live much longer for the old style diet is a killer.

These are not just sensational words for effect but the message from the British government's National Advisory Committee on Nutrition Education, 1981's most recent report on the nation's diet and health. The report states that anyone who eats the average western diet is in grave danger. We eat far too much food stuffed with calories and rich in fat. Too much fat leads to high cholesterol levels leading to heart disease, which kills twice as many people in western countries each year as cancer and 25 times as many as road accidents. It is the biggest killer of men over 40.

Obviously there are many factors relating to heart disease apart from diet, as we shall see in chapter 14, but if we start eating the right foods we are well on the way to delaying the degenerative diseases of the

arteries. And we are well on the way towards having some of that zes
for life and vital energy we all would like.

A vegetarian diet

The trouble with the Western-style diet is that we are not eating
enough of the foods that keep us young, and eating too much of those
that age us. We must eat many more fresh vegetables and fruits. In fact
there is much to be said for the vegetarian diet, if we heed recent
medical inquiries.

In California two doctors have carefully monitored the health of a
group of people for the last 20 years — a large community of Seventh
Day Adventists. Half of these live on a vegetarian diet that also
includes eggs and dairy products. The study shows that the
vegetarians living in that community with exactly the same way of life
in every other respect, are half as likely to develop cancer of the bowel
as other Americans. They also have lower rates of cancer of the ovary,
breast, pancreas and prostate. That would seem a convincing case in
itself. But there is more. Research into this vegetarian group also
showed that middle-aged men who regularly eat meat are four times as
likely to die of heart attack than non-meat-eaters.

More evidence comes to light every day about the benefits of a
vegetarian diet. In Israel a survey showed that only two per cent of
vegetarians suffered from high blood pressure. And in Finland, where
a high incidence of heart disease had caused a switch of diet from
butter and dairy products to a vegetarian diet, there followed a
remarkable drop in the number of heart attacks.

Now, before you switch your dietary habits to completely vegetarian
ones, there is a word of warning. Do not replace meat with a lot of
bread, butter and cheese. Go easy on the high fat dairy products.
Another point to bear in mind when balancing the arguments for and
against a vegetarian diet is that although reports suggest that
vegetarians, generally speaking, are more healthy than meat eaters,
many people would say that their own day to day experience does not
support the idea and that the likely reason that vegetarians are found
by research doctors to be healthier is that vegetarians are by nature
more concerned about their habits affecting their health across the
whole spectrum.

Perhaps it would be wise to keep everything in perspective. It would be a pity to deny ourselves the enjoyment of roast beef altogether. There is probably a place for everything, a juicy steak occasionally and a good proportion of fresh vegetables and salads. And when on this subject we should not forget the special merits of garlic and onions. They not only enhance the flavour of foods but help to keep you healthy.

Garlic

Garlic, traditionally hung up in horror films to ward off vampires, can also help to ward off infections, heart disease, and high blood pressure. Medical scientists now probing its folk use as a medicine have come to the conclusion that it has remarkable health-giving properties. For centuries gypsies have gathered wild garlic to treat their families and sick animals. It is said to make hair grow thicker and glossier and that it helps to cure chest complaints. There are stories of how garlic was rubbed on wounds in World War 1 to prevent gangrene, and was thought long ago to aid circulation. According to folklore garlic makes the blood flow easier.

In the history of medical practice, garlic is featured constantly as a remedy for a wide range of ailments. Louis Pasteur was using it as an antiseptic in 1858 and now research at Harvard University suggests that one of garlic's properties can stop the spread of cancerous growths. Other reports indicate that regular use of garlic in food can lower cholesterol levels in the blood thus reducing the risk of heart disease.

Scientists have found a chemical in garlic called 'ajoene' which they believe holds the clue to its beneficial properties. The compound may be useful as a blood thinner in the treatment of numerous circulatory ailments. For those who do not care for the stong smell of garlic on the breath, there are garlic pearls – capsules which are just as effective but less anti-social.

Onions, too, from ancient times are known for mystical medicinal powers. Modern research now brings evidence to support their use in meals. They also can help to lower cholesterol levels and so play a part in the prevention of heart disease. Eat them raw or cooked for they contain many important nutrients – folate, iron, calcium, potassium and vitamin A.

14

The eating for health diet

What is becoming abundantly clear today is that a well planned, nutritious diet keeps the body vibrantly fit for a full life. This demands a little thought on your part. You cannot expect to make do on convenience foods and still not pay the penalty in terms of ageing. Poorly fed people — underweight and overweight — are likely to have that chronically tired look that goes with the unfit and the elderly. But this does not mean that you have to stick to a monotonously strict routine of 'healthy' foods. Far from it. Your meals should be enjoyable catering for individual tastes within the basic guidelines set out below. Another basic principle is to eat as wide a variety of foods as possible. This should ensure that if one particular nutrient is deficient it could be made up by an excess of another, provided it is more or less in the same food group.

If you include in your diet a portion of food from each of the groups listed below then you can be sure of having a well balanced diet. (See also main meal suggestions on pages 134 to 137, Appendix II.)

GROUP ONE

Meat and fish, chicken, shell fish, liver and eggs

These are 'building' foods that can be interchanged for variety. Liver is real value-for-money food, rich in iron and vitamins, and excellent in protein too.

GROUP TWO

Dairy products, milk, cheese yoghurt

These are also building foods, proteins needed for repair of tissue, strong muscles and energy. Take care not to have too much of full fat cream cheeses which are high in energy and might be stored as fat.

GROUP THREE

Cereals, oats, wholemeal bread, rice, peas and beans, nuts

These are the cheapest and simplest of energy foods. We have a bonus in bread of being a good source of vitamin B1. Wholegrain pastas, breakfast cereals and bread make good 'roughage' too.

GROUP FOUR

Margarine, cooking oils, salad oils, oily fish like herrings and mackerel, sardines

These are good energy foods, and a good source of vitamin D. They are inexpensive foods that give us vitamin D as well as body-building protein.

GROUP FIVE

Vegetables, root and leafy, fresh fruit

Most of these provide their maximum nutrition when eaten raw. Otherwise lightly cooked is recommended. As you cannot store vitamins in the body you need a supply daily. You need the vitamin C that is in one orange, or half a grapefruit, or three boiled potatoes daily. Not all fruits are rich in vitamin C – you would need 12 pears to get what you can get from one orange. Citrus fruits and berries and green vegetables are the richest source.

To take full responsibility for your own eating habits, bearing in mind the warnings of the government report, you just have to spend a little time in planning what changes have to be made so that you can avoid the hazards and reap the benefits of a more beneficial vegetarian-type diet.

Eat less fat

Countries that eat a lot of fat have the highest incidence of heart disease. Avoid animal fats – even lean meat has more fat tucked away between the muscle fibres than is evident upon first inspection, so trimming away what we can see does not solve the problem. Pies, pastry, sausages, bacon, salami, mayonnaise, potato crisps (chips), cream filled chocolates, gateaux and full-fat cheese have a high percentage of fat in them.

Unfortunately this is not all the story about fat. When we eat too much, our Calorie intake is high, and even carbohydrates are all too readily converted into fat in the body. So we not only need to eat less fat but we need generally to eat less, too.

Eat less sugar

'Pure, white and deadly' is how it has been described.

Only about half the sugar we eat comes directly from the packet. The other half comes largely from the sugar added to processed foods. Look on the wrappers and labels and you will find sugar mentioned in the ingredients of a surprising number of preparations such as baked beans, sweet corn, sauces such as Bolognese, and chilli con carne, tinned soups and chicken dishes.

For years we have been conditioned to expect sugar as an added piquancy in our foods and we have grown up with the idea that because sugar provides a lot of Calories then the food must be nourishing. This is not true. The Calories are 'empty' Calories providing energy fuel but no vitamins or minerals. If you fill up on sugary foods because you feel satisfied after eating them you will not be eating enough of the nutritious foods. You will be over-fed but under-nourished.

Eat less salt

Most of us eat more than 10 times the amount of salt that we need. Some is necessary as a regulator of the body processes but we certainly do not need all that we consume and the excess is contributing to our premature ageing and earlier deaths.

High salt-eating populations such as the British, have far more people who suffer from high blood pressure which can lead to heart attacks and strokes.

Do not add salt to food before cooking, is the advice both doctors and nutrition experts now give. Do not pour salt onto food before you taste it. For piquancy, a little lemon juice is a useful substitute.

Eat more fibre

The type of diet least likely to cause disease is one that provides a high proportion of Calories in whole grain, cereals, vegetables and fruit. These foods have a high fibre content. Sprinkling bran on all your dishes is not enough, and too much bran is not good for you. Fibre passes through the digestive and excretory systems as roughage. By holding water as it passes through the bowel it keeps the motion soft and bulky thus speeding the flow of the food, helping to prevent many disorders of the bowel apart from constipation. Studies of the diet of African tribes who live mainly on vegetables and fruit have shown that there is a very much lower incidence of cancer of the bowel there than in Europe.

It is not just the foods that seem crunchy and stringy that are high in fibre − bananas, for example, have just as much fibre as an apple. Dried fruits are particularly recommended, apricots are especially high in fibre content. Buy them dried, chop them and add them to muesli for breakfast.

A glance at the fibre chart at the end of the book will show some of the relatively high fibre foods that can easily be brought into everyday diet. Potatoes are good for you particularly with their skins on. Three medium sized old potatoes boiled have as much vitamin C as one orange, and they are a good source of energy fuel. Figs, prunes, pulses of all kinds − especially of the bean family − and nuts, are most beneficial in a rejuvenating diet programme.

Make sure of your vitamin intake

We all know that vitamins are essential for good health. We also know that nutrition specialists often tell us in no uncertain terms that vitamin pills are largely a waste of money and we'd be better off healthwise and financially using the money to buy fresh foods which have all the right vitamins. As John Yudkin, Emeritus Professor of Nutrition at London University, tells us, taking too many vitamins in pill form can be harmful. OK − if you *are* eating a well balanced diet. But who is? Are the millions of people who live on their own eating 'meat and two veg' dinners? Are all the overworked single parent family Mums (and Dads)? Are those who do not know and don't have enough money or time? Perhaps not.

One thing we do know is that another report tells us that millions of people in the Western industrialised countries are already living off diets deficient in essential vitamins and minerals. For example, when whole grains are milled into flour they lose almost 75 per cent of vitamin B6 and nearly 90 per cent of their vitamin E. Yes, we could get all our nutrition from good whole, fresh food but we would often need to eat more in terms of Calories than we actually want. Furthermore, we should never be sure of the nutritional value of meals we eat out in restaurants.

To be sure, then, there is a strong argument for taking a supplementary ration of vitamins as pills, if we are in any doubt and if we can afford the cost. For those who would prefer to shop around for the right foods here is a quick guide.

VITAMIN A:	Offal such as kidneys, liver and hearts; vegetables such as marrow, carrots and green leaf vegetables.
VITAMIN B:	Whole grains, brewer's yeast, nuts, eggs and liver.
VITAMIN C:	Rose hips, citrus fruits, green peppers, broccoli, watercress, parsley, potatoes (especially when eaten without being peeled).
VITAMIN D:	We manufacture much of our own vitamin D from sunlight on the skin provided we get enough sunshine. Asians in Britain have been found to need extra vitamin D. It is found in fish oils, sardines, herrings, mackerel, sunflower seeds, eggs and milk.
VITAMIN E:	A useful vitamin which can help to slow down the ageing process. Found in sprouting seeds, almonds, walnuts, spinach and eggs.
VITAMIN F:	Very fresh vegetables, and sprouting seeds.
VITAMIN K:	Mainly from fresh green leaves of plants.

Special needs

Women who are pregnant or breast feeding need to take special care with vitamin intake. Other conditions in which extra supplements of vitamins are recommended are Pre-Menstrual Tension – PMT – and the depression sometimes associated with the pill.

Another way of checking your intake is to look at the foods which would give you a weekly supply of essential vitamins. They are listed below.

Bread, whole grain and whole grain cereals.
Dairy products, skimmed milk, cottage cheese and yoghurt.
Lean meat – fat trimmed away, twice a week is enough.
Liver – once a week or fortnight in addition to meat.
White Meat – poultry twice a week.
White Fish – once or twice a week.
Oily Fish – mackerel, sardines, herrings twice a week.
Fresh raw fruit – eat without peeling as often as possible.
Fresh leafy green vegetables – or frozen ones can be just as good, frequently.
Low cholesterol margarine – better for you than butter.

More and more people are becoming vegetarian, not in a fastidious way but simply because they are beginning to realise the advantages of eating vegetables more often than they used to. They say they feel better for it. And they tell each other. There is nothing quite like the word of mouth recommendation — especially when it comes with bright-eyed, healthy enthusiasm for the abundant energy and the leaner look that vegetarians often have. And there is a lot more to be said for that lean look.

To summarise

1) Get away from the traditional heart-disease diet.
2) Fresh fruit, fresh vegetables and high fibre are the watchwords for a healthy diet.
3) Fast foods often lack essential vitamins.
4) You are what you eat.

3 GET THE LEAN LOOK

'Once you get to my age you can't avoid thinking about time,' said Paul Newman. 'When I was 20 it took about a year for a year to go by. Now a year goes by in two and a half months.' Incredibly, the handsome man with the lean look and the boyish mischievous grin celebrated his 60th birthday still looking a good 10 to 15 years younger.

It certainly pays dividends to keep that lean look. But time tends to pass more quickly, as Paul Newman pointed out, and we have none to waste when we are responsible for the upkeep, and servicing of our own bodies. It is far easier to keep lean and slim than to take off the flab once you have let it build up with the passing years. Getting rid of excess weight is a problem that only a few solve.

Every year 60 per cent of men and women try to lose weight; and predictably only 5 per cent, we are told, succeed in sustaining their weight loss. Consequently there is a continuous flow of new diets from the press and television. There must now be as many slimming diets as flakes in a muesli mixture. For dieting is really big business.

Some of the diets become more fashionable than others because of the gimmick appeal which catches the gullible. It might be an alliterative title that trips off the tongue − like the 'bran and banana diet', or the 'paw-paw and pineapple'; or it could be an intriguing title that sounds more like a Secret Service Code than a simple slimming system. Quite often the diets recommended are not based on scientific principles − such as the 'fat eats fat' variety − and could be more likely to lead to ill health than beneficial weight loss. How could anyone hope to select the best diet from all these? Are they all effective? If so, why do so many people on these diets fail to sustain their weight loss? Ask around your friends and they'll tell you the same sad story.

There is one good reason why they fail. And it is this. Diets do not work until they get to the root of the problem posed by the questions: 'Why do people get fat?' and 'Why do these people continue to eat more than they need when they know for sure that they are overweight and can no longer get into the clothes they used to wear?'. 'Why do they carry so much extra weight that they can no longer do all the things they used to do easily?' And why do they deliberately make themselves ugly? These questions must be answered honestly. Then a sensible diet will work.

After all these years of public interest in the subject and scientific research, there is a definitive way of dieting. It has no gimmicks, but it works. We'll come to it shortly – the short term 'hospital' diet and the long term sequel. But meanwhile let us look at those questions a little more closely.

Why do people get fat?

'It's no use talking to me about diets. They have absolutely no effect on me. It's my glands!' You've heard it said no doubt. It's rubbish! Continual overeating is the cause of 90 per cent of all cases of being overweight. Only rarely is the condition attributable to inactivity of the ductless glands – thyroid, pituitary or sex glands, nor can excessive weight usually be attributed to fluid retention. Professor Yudkin writes: 'If you are overweight but otherwise healthy, then I'm afraid that what you are retaining is not fluid – it's fat.' (*A-Z of Slimming*, Davis-Poynter, London 1977).

The compulsion to eat more and more of the wrong foods is due to a complex mesh of feelings and fears. Psychologists say that overeating sometimes is a form of compensation for emotional insecurity or frustration. Women who fear the loss of their husband's love, men who are frustrated in their ambitions, children of unhappy parents, find solace in eating more than they need. For them, food symbolises security. It has even been reported that men can allow themselves to get grossly fat because of fear of impotence, reasoning that if they look so unappealing no one will try to seduce them.

An easily accepted reason for both men and women becoming overweight is that the healthy appetite of a sportingly energetic youth has been retained into the less active 30s. That and the faded sports shirt, a photograph and a dusty long-unused tennis racquet being the only things that remain of their sporting days. The food that once used to feed the active muscles is no longer burnt in vigorous effort on the sports field or tennis court. It is stored between the wasting muscle fibres as useless fat.

Eating habits are hard to break especially when, during the more prosperous years of the late 20s and early 30s, a little extra money is available for gratifying the pleasures of eating rich meals. And though such extra treats may only add two or three pounds to body weight in one year, it can at that rate easily creep up to an unhealthy stone in five years.

Many doctors place the blame for excess weight on the parents of young children, for their outdated idea that children ought to be 'fat and bonny'. Fat children are now a serious medical problem, says Dr Ann Mullins, an authority on children's health. She writes that in boys and girls of all ages overweight goes with more diseases and higher death rate. Parents of the fat child may console themselves by saying: 'It's only puppy fat and he'll grow out of it,' but only a few fat children lose their excess weight without positive direction and help with their eating habits. Fat children grow into fat adults. They are burdened with a lifetime of ill-health and psychological complications.

Consider your own case now. When did you first begin to get fatter? Is there a cause you can eliminate? If yours is a psychological craving a substitute should be found, or if your eating habits seem to have been bad, revise them. When the cause is understood, the cure is easier to undertake.

Now what is the task facing the slimmer? How many pounds need to be shed?

What is your ideal weight?

The usual definition of your ideal weight is the weight on your 25th birthday, and for most people this would be true. But in other instances, perhaps because of illness, malnutrition or unusual circumstances, the weight at 25 might not have been the right one. To define accurate ideal weights for age and height is also difficult because body types for both men and women vary. Some have big bones and a large frame to cover with muscle and fatty tissue. Others, of similar height, have smaller skeletal frames. Consequently, on the chart showing ideal weights for size and age an allowance of 10 per cent either way can be made for different body types.

To be absolutely sure − and if you are worried about whether you are carrying too much fat or not − ask your doctor for guidance. Only he can tell accurately what you ought to weigh by comparing your body type with detailed medical charts for average heights and weights.

How much weight do you need to lose?

You don't need to look fat to be overweight. Excess poundage can creep on insidiously with the passing years and can become a threat to your health. So you could be overweight without realising it. Shedding this excess in your prime would bring a level of well-being and vitality which you have long forgotten, or have never previously enjoyed.

Try these tests:

1) Is it harder for you now to squeeze into clothes you cast off years ago?
2) Does your flesh ripple and joggle as you bounce up and down. Look in a full length mirror and be prepared for a shock.
3) Pinch the flesh on the back of your upper arm mid-way between your shoulder and elbow. If it's more than an inch thick you're far too fat.

Use the Guide to Calorie Requirements for Women and Men below as an approximate guide to what you should eat, and the Ideal Weight Chart in Appendix V.

There is no crash diet that works! Furthermore, the quick weight loss diets are dangerous. A daily 1,000 Calorie diet is normally recommended as the safe low-Calorie level for weight reducing. Avoid diets claiming an initial weight loss of ten pounds a week for the first two weeks. You will feel dreadful and look awful for the fortnight of deprivation. These diets are usually very low in Calories from carbohydrates and high in proteins. Some of these diets involve eating more eggs than is good for health − they are rich in cholesterol, a cause of heart disease. No more than three eggs a week is recommended.

A diet in one best selling guide depends upon eating little else but

GUIDE TO CALORIE REQUIREMENTS FOR WOMEN AND MEN

(a) For those not engaged in physically hard work (sedentary occupations)

Women

Build	20 to 40 years	40 to 50 years	50 plus
9st Small	2000	1900	1800
10st Medium	2200	2100	2000
11st Large	2400	2300	2200

Men

	20 to 40 years	40 to 50 years	50 plus
10½st Small	2500	2400	2300
11½st Medium	2700	2600	2400
13½st Large	3000	2600	2400

(b) For those working hard physically

Women

	20 to 40 years	40 to 50 years	50 plus
9st Small	2200	2100	2000
10st Medium	2300	2200	2100
11st Large	2700	2500	2400

Men

	20 to 40 years	40 to 50 years	50 plus
10½st Small	2700	2600	2500
11½st Medium	2900	2800	2600
13½st Large	3300	3100	3000

fruit for the first ten days and much is made of the magic properties of combining certain foods, as if eating certain foods together facilitates weight loss. There is no scientific foundation for this theory. No magic in it either. Any weight you might lose on such a diet would be simply because you are taking in fewer Calories than you are expending in energy. Sudden weight loss on these crash diets leaves you often with that skin-sagging tired look of the undernourished.

Hospital 1,000 Calorie slimming diet

There are times when you go to your doctor for one purpose and find that you are referred to a hospital for further tests. And it often happens that one of the first things you have to do is to lose weight.

You could be put on to this 1,000 Calorie diet which a neighbour of mine was handed with strict instructions to follow it and nothing else.

'You have to forget all other advice and keep to this diet,' he was told, 'And come back in four weeks' time to be weighed.'

This was his daily allowance:

Milk — ½ pint (250ml)
Margarine — ½ oz (15g)
Bread — 3 slices

BREAKFAST
Small bowl of porridge or other cereal
Half a grapefruit
White fish — 4 oz (125g), or an egg

MID-MORNING BREAK
Tea or meat or yeast extract drink
No sugar or squash drink

MIDDAY
Clear soup
Meat — 2 oz (60g), or cheese — 1 oz (30g), or fish — 5 oz (150g)
Potatoes — 4 oz (125g)
Green vegetables or salad — a large helping
Broad beans — a tablespoon (20ml)
Tea or coffee

DINNER
Clear soup
Meat — 2 oz (60g), or fish — 5 oz (150g)
Green vegetables or salad — a large helping
Fruit — raw, fresh, or stewed without sugar
Tea or coffee

With this diet the pounds dropped off dramatically. Obviously it is not the sort of diet you would like to keep on for a long time. Once your weight is down to a healthy level then you should maintain it by a more varied diet which follows the principles of the healthy food diet explained below.

The healthy food diet

There is no gimmick, no punishment, and no sacrifice. Consequently it might have little popular appeal. But it works! Weight reduction can be achieved without much hardship or need for stoic willpower. Provided meals are prepared from low-Calorie foods, satisfying and bulky helpings can be enjoyed. On the healthy food diet you will steadily lose weight until you have reached the plateau of your natural weight. And you will not regain the excess you were carrying before you changed your eating habits.

Once you embark upon this effective diet, the first requirement is to stop reading other articles upon the subject because you remember snippets from a confusing mass of material such as: 'Eat as much as you like of . . .' and 'some people eat far too little on slimming diets and they would lose at least as much weight, if not more, just as quickly on a higher Calorie intake . . .' And they use these snippets as an excuse for having a little more far too often.

Stick to one system: the healthy food diet. There are no taboo foods, but those that are fattening should only be eaten most infrequently and as a special treat. Before you start your new diet stock your pantry with non-fattening foods. And also have something readily available for those times when you might just be feeling a little bit hungry and yet have a few Calories left from your daily ration; the following are recommended: raw carrot, sticks of celery, pears, home-made clear soup.

Cut your intake of fat by half – use less margarine spread on bread, (sunflower margarine high in polyunsaturates and low in cholesterol is better for you than butter) avoid cream cheeses and full fat milk. You can have all the nutritional benefits of milk – the wide variety of minerals and vitamins without the fat, from skimmed milk.

If you make really good, home baked, wholemeal bread it is so tasty that you will enjoy eating it without having to spread anything on it. It's easier to make than you might think.

Do not add salt to your cooking – use herbs to add flavour instead. Eat potatoes in their skin – it's a good source of fibre and vitamins, boiled or baked. Cut down on all sugar, avoid the excessively refined processed foods and sweetened drinks. You can still drink beer and wine but remember that it takes half a pound of sugar to make a bottle of wine!

Have bowls of fruit about the house and even in the car. And get used to the idea that a third or second course of pudding or sweet desserts is not a necessary complement to the main meal course.

Follow the sensible eating habits outlined above and you will soon have no appetite at all for the fatty and processed foods you used to eat. The healthy food diet will then have become a lifetime habit. Not only will you be slimmer and healthier but you will look ten years younger than you would have done had you retained the unhealthy habits of eating which far too many of us have had in the past. And that is not altogether our fault. For too long, we have been conditioned into eating the wrong foods, and the situation is getting worse. In schools today the meal service is encouraging bad eating habits. In going over to fast foods and a cafeteria system the traditional 'meat and two veg' course has been driven out in favour of pasties, burgers, sausages, chips, baked beans and sweet puddings. Take this recipe for example, as a tasty treat for school dinner: ½lb (250g) margarine, ½lb (250g) lard, ½lb (250g) icing sugar, 1lb (500g) of soft flour and a dot of jam. This is the recipe for 30 Viennese shortcakes for 30 schoolchildren. A 'firm favourite' in Derbyshire schools, says the local education authority. It is also a recipe for disaster. A recipe which would turn the stomach of any self-respecting health food fan.

Anyone wishing to keep slim today has a lot to fight against. We are bombarded with advertisements for foods that are unhealthy. How can the Health Education Council compete with the millions spent on creating a demand for fatty and sugary foods?

Fortunately the situation is not all gloom. A bright ray of hope comes from some of the well-known supermarkets which are now labelling their products clearly to show the fat and sugar content. And slowly our eating habits are changing. Countries are campaigning in various ways to stop people killing themselves with food. One Australian television sequence shows a young man and a girl savouring succulent fruit, juice flowing down their chins as they eye each other lasciviously. Their thoughts are clearly on other things than the fruit. The film ends abruptly with the words: 'That's the way to get it off. Eat fruit instead of fat.' Good advice indeed.

Eight golden rules for the healthy food diet

1) Drink plenty. Dehydrating is nonsense.

2) Moderate alcohol. The body uses alcohol as a source of energy. Food taken in meals is thus left free for storing as fat. One pint of beer has the same Calorific value as two eggs.
3) Skim fat from soups. This is best done by storing overnight in the fridge when the hardened fat is more easily taken off.
4) Eat less red meat. Take skin, with its layer of fat, from chicken.
5) Always eat breakfast. If you do not you will be more tempted to overeat later in the day.
6) One meal a day must be very light. This ensures a low Calorie intake. Lunch is probably the best meal to skimp. You can then eat a more normal meal with your family and friends in the evening.
7) Take halibut or cod liver oil tablets every other day if you feel that you are not having enough of the fat soluble vitamins from your fat free diet.
8) Weigh yourself weekly at the same time in the early morning, without clothes. Make a note of your weight on a card kept near the scales. Most people weigh more late at night than they do just before breakfast.

Shaping up

In a well planned attack through diet and exercise, weight can drop quickly, giving the body a severe shock. So, monitor your weight and efforts carefully.

Losses at first will depend upon how overweight you are, the rigorous nature of the exercise taken, and the limitations of the food intake. Do not be surprised to find a drop of 3kg (7 lbs) in the first week. Not all of this will be fat – there will be some water shed. After this there will be a more gradual loss until a plateau is reached as the body adjusts to the new regime. To drop below this plateau, a change in the campaign is sometimes necessary – a stricter control of food intake and an increase in physical activity might be needed so as to overcome the way that the body, by becoming more efficient in utilising food, has adjusted to the drop in energy fuel and increase in work load. Such a change will cause weight to drop again gradually.

Loss of fat from the body

Men like fat to go from the waistline, and women like it to go from the hips. In the first week both could be disappointed. The body can be perverse in the way that it uses up its stock of fat. Those body parts which are the first to show an increase of weight are often the last to lose it. Hence it is important to persevere with the programme until a complete re-adjustment has been made.

Do not be surprised then, at the first alteration in body proportions, they will come right soon enough. Women with a small bust are sometimes shocked to find diet and exercise has shrunk it even smaller. They can take heart, for the 'press away' exercise of the training circuit develops the pectoral muscles which lie under the breasts. Through progressive resistance exercise the fibres of these muscles become broader and new capillaries open up to feed the muscles. The increased blood supply carries vital energy fuel and tissue building material to the working muscle and so a new form begins to take shape. It is a more healthy form, firmer, built naturally from new muscle tissue and a little fat.

Similarly men may find that the initial loss of fat from the face and neck will give them a leaner look to begin with whilst the waistband tightness has altered little; just as the woman with broad hips and fat thighs may find these areas show little change at first despite a real drop in body weight. Have faith! After a few weeks the body proportions will return to what they were before the fat tide came in. And everybody will be delighted with the new shape – everybody that is, except your fat and envious friends.

Keeping a youthful figure

You've seen it happen, I'm sure. A steady weight loss in someone at work; new clothes, new style of hair, a new image. Smirks of self-righteous satisfaction from the slimmer one, mixed response from her colleagues.

What happens next? Statistics say that most slip back to former eating habits and over indulgence in food. The pounds creep back on. But there is no need to return to old ways and their ageing effect on the figure and movement. Part of your slimming programme must involve building a new way of life where new habits work for you without any conscious thought or effort on your part. They should become second nature to you. Your body weight will then fluctuate very little.

But just to make sure, keep your ideal weight target clear in your mind, literally branded upon your chest if you like, in clear figures so that when you weigh yourself each weekend you will know immediately if you are straying over this boundary mark. Immediately you find this happening then take corrective action, reduce food intake and increase the exercise stint. Once you have felt the boost that the leaner look gives to your life then hold on to it. Keep that waistline trim. If those measurements begin to creep up to chest measurements then you are in real trouble. A formidable health hazard. Keep that tum flat!

To summarise

1) Keeping slim and trim is easier than shedding weight later.
2) Crash diets invariably fail. They do not keep you slim: avoid them.
3) Work out why you have been eating more than you need.
4) Be clear in your aims. Know why you want to be slimmer.
5) Aim for your ideal weight by setting a target for each month. Consult the weight charts.
6) Keep to the healthy food diet. Use the 'hospital' diet only for the initial period.
7) Weigh yourself regularly.

4 FLATTEN THAT TUM!

It was just before curtain time. The Opera House was a forest of flowers, the audience dressed to the teeth and bejewelled to blind the eye. An aura of excitement hung over the auditorium, but backstage hostility was in the air. Waiting to make her debut in the title role of Puccini's *Tosca* was a raven-haired overweight soprano.

Stage lights brightened, tongues ran swiftly round drying lips, deep breaths were taken. And it was then, from backstage, that a loud voice rang out. 'That fat bitch will never carry it off!'

Never did such a magnificent career have such a daunting beginning. But Maria Callas, one of the world's greatest operatic singers had learnt a hard lesson. She knew she was fat. In her own eyes, 'An ugly duckling, fat, clumsy and unloved.' She grew up tortured by fears and doubts, painfully aware of her parent's disappointment that she had been born a girl when they had so desperately yearned for a boy, rankled by jealousy of her more favoured sister. And for consolation she stuffed herself with food.

By the time she came to London for the first time she weighed 15 stone. Her voice stunned enraptured audiences and her performances were acclaimed with prolonged ovations. Despite this reception she was sensitive to a major defect – the difficulty a woman so massive has in portraying a girlish lover.

She tackled the problem with the determination of one who is motivated with a desperate need to succeed. It was a task most women would have declared beyond hope. And this is why I mention it now. In 12 months she transformed herself dramatically from a 15 stone heavyweight to a 10 stone elegant beauty. She lost 5 stone.

Her spectacular weight loss came in for a round of questioning. What was the secret? An Italian spaghetti firm claimed in advertisements that the amazing slimming feat was achieved by a steady diet of Pantanella's 'psychological macaroni', others attributed it to a glandular disturbance which had rectified itself. Maria herself said, 'Heavens, if I had a reducing system I would not keep it a secret. I could become the richest woman in the world.'

There was no secret really. She was successful, happy and in love. Gone was the need to eat for consolation. Furthermore she was aware that opera is a fiercely competitive business and Maria Callas had always been a fierce competitor for nothing came easily to her.

Once she had triumphed over the weight problem she was freed from her most painful inhibitions. She went from success to success. It had been worth all the effort.

Flattening that tum can be worth a lot to everyone. Nothing ages you so much as when the flat teenage waistline goes to pot and a spare tyre rests where it should not be. It immediately gives the stamp of middle age. Remove the inches, you will feel fitter and look younger.

A protruding paunch, though, is not merely an embarrassment. It is a hazard to health. Medical evidence shows that when waistline measurements exceed those of the fully expanded chest by more than 2 inches, the mortality risk increases by 50 per cent above that calculated for the overweight condition itself. The disproportionate excess by inches is just as important as the excessive poundage. It pays to flatten the stomach. You will live longer, and the guy in your life (or the lady) will love you that bit more.

How the paunch develops

Just as little acorns grow into great oaks, so little pots have a nasty habit of growing into bigger pots. We can flatten the stomach better when we understand what has been going on beneath that disfiguring paunch.

The stomach, liver, small intestine and other abdominal organs are carried in the bowl-shaped cavity of the pelvis. All these organs are attached to the rear surface of the bowl by loose connective tissue. The back and sides of this bowl-shaped container are formed by the bones of the pelvis. The front is the weakest part for it is not bone but muscle which can be stretched. If the pelvis is tilted forward, because of a hollow back, the abdominal contents slip forward and lie heavily against the front muscular wall of the bowl.

The constant drag of the fluid-filled intestines in time stretches the tissue which attaches them to the spine at the rear until eventually the whole weight of the intestines flops entirely on the inadequate muscular wall, which is far too weak to carry the extra burden. Consequently the abdominal muscles sag and the contents of the abdomen slip still further forward instead of lying snugly in their proper place.

Many doctors say this displacement impairs efficient functioning. It can be the cause of nervous irritation, digestive disorders, and inflammatory conditions. Furthermore, when the muscle fibres of the abdomen are weak there is an increased susceptibility to hernia. But worse conditions can follow.

When the abdominal wall muscles lose their natural tone and droop you become liable to suffering from one of the most common afflications of our times — back-ache. You need strong abdominal muscles to support the lower segments of the spine. It is the pull of the three main muscle groups of the abdomen that holds the pelvis in position, preventing the lower part of the spine from falling forward. And when this happens the alignment of the spine is altered so that the cushioning discs between each vertebra are compressed in a different manner. In time these discs can 'slip' and press against nerves, causing pain in the back and down the leg.

To ensure against back pain and sciatica later in life you have to keep your stomach muscles trim by exercise and habitual good posture. In fact, one of the prime causes of a paunch is poor posture in both sitting and standing. When we slump in a chair at a desk or when driving a car, the spine does not do its fair share in supporting the weight of the chest and head. Instead all this weight rests practically unsupported on the abdomen and the effect is similar to placing a heavy load on a balloon — as its height is diminished the balloon bulges outwards. When the abdominal cavity is compressed, the contents are forced against the resilient front muscle wall which eventually gives way and sags under the continual strain.

In a good sitting posture the spine holds the body erect and the height of the abdomen is not diminished. The pressure is thus taken off the distended stomach muscles.

You can remove inches from your waist measurement in a very simple way which has an immediate effect. All you need to do is to straighten the shoulders, push the top of your head towards the sky and lift the rib cage. You have probably done it scores of times after catching sight of your profile in a full-length mirror and you automatically brace up. For a few weeks make a definite effort to be

34

aware of your posture in sitting, standing and walking; tuck in your waistline and walk 'tall'. Flattening the stomach will then be merely a matter of therapeutic exercise and diet. Exercise removes the inches and diet the pounds.

It is not going to be easy at first. But it can be done and you will see the rejuvenating effects of the trimming process within a month. The annoying feature of this process is that for most people the abdomen is the very first place to accumulate fat and the last to release it, as we have already noted in a previous chapter.

What we have to do is to restore to the weakened abdominal muscles their former length and strength, and to improve the tone of the dorsal muscles, needed for good posture. But take care. Some of the exercises often prescribed as 'tummy trimmers' do more harm than good. For example, one of the exercises which frequently illustrates a reducing regime is the one in which both legs are raised and lowered from the back-lying position. Yet this exercise has been condemned for years by physiotherapists. It is mainly an exercise for the hip muscles and can have a harmful effect upon weakened abdominals working hard trying to maintain the fixed position for the exercise. Professor Katherine Wells writes: 'This is an exercise which only those who already have strong abdominals should be permitted to do, and then only with the most careful supervision.'

Not so harmful but equally futile is an exercise often recommended for 'whittling the waistline' – legs astride, alternate toe touching.

Unfortunately, most popular physical recreational activities such as cycling, squash, and jogging, do not even begin to strengthen the muscles of the abdominal wall in such a way as would have any effect on the waistline other than from burning up fat. What is needed is a special rehabilitation exercise routine for the three abdominal muscles: the rectus abdomis, the external and internal obliques, and the transversalis. (See Figures 3–5.)

The long column of muscle running from the breast bone to the pubis (rectus abdominis) comes into action when the trunk is flexed at the waist. The oblique muscles running 'V' shaped across the abdomen in the way that corset manufacturers try to imitate, are used to twist the trunk and hold the abdomen compactly. A broad flat sheet of muscle (the transversalis) lying deeply below the other layers of muscle runs horizontally across the body and compresses the abdominal contents. It comes into action when you are trying to look

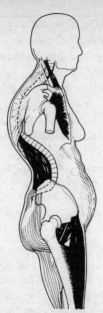

Fig. 1   Diagram showing the unbalanced development of the postural muscles associated with a sagging stomach and round back. The weak and elongated muscles are slightly shaded, the short and more powerful ones are shown in black. Notice how the pelvis is tilted forward because of the hollowing of the back and weakened front wall of the abdomen

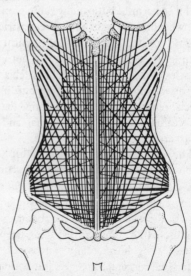

Fig. 2   Muscles of the abdomen

your best on the beach or side of the swimming pool with your abdomen pulled in and chest out.

The special exercises that follow will help to keep all these important muscles strong and in good shape for years to come.

Stomach flattening exercises

For the rectus abdominis which controls the tilt of the pelvis
Trunk curl with bent knee
Lie flat on the floor, bend the knees slightly. Curl the body forward and reach forward with your hands to let them slide over the tops of the knees. Do as many repetitions as you can with comfort and without strain. Rest a few moments and then repeat. Count the number of repetitions and note your score so that you can measure progress.

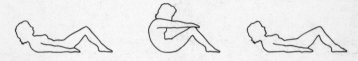

Fig. 3   Trunk-curl with bent knee

For the external and internal oblique muscles which compress the stomach
Trunk twisting and lowering backwards
Sit on the floor with the legs comfortably apart. Turn to look behind you as far as you can without undue strain and lower your trunk to the ground. Repeat, turning to the other side. Alternate from side to side until you have completed as many movements as possible. Do not worry if you cannot get far round and do not force your trunk round more than you can do comfortably.

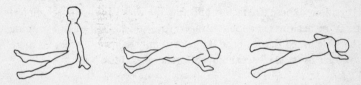

Fig. 4   Trunk twisting and lowering backwards

For the transversalis muscle which helps to hold the stomach in
Abdominal retraction

This is not an easy movement for some people. It takes a little practice, for the technique of 'sucking the stomach in' to be learnt. To begin, stand with your hands on your thighs, shoulders rounded forward and body leaning slightly forward at the hips. Breathe out forcibly, and pull in your stomach. Practise the movement at odd times during the day.

In this movement the transversalis muscle works against the weight of the intestines. It develops broader and thicker fibres in the transversalis muscle to cope with this weight in the exercise in the same way that biceps develop in performing the arm curl exercise with dumb-bells. Eventually the abdominal muscles will be strong and short enough to hold your slimmer paunch back in its original position, leaving you with a teenage flat stomach.

Fig. 5   Abdominal retraction

To summarise

The routine to flatten the stomach should include:

1) A reducing diet.
2) General exercises to burn Calories stored as fat.
3) Specific exercises to rehabilitate the abdominal muscles.
4) Strengthening exercises for the back and shoulder muscles.
5) Constant re-education of the feeling for good posture.

Attention to these five factors affecting the waistline can make you feel fitter, be healthier and look younger. And you are half way to winning that celebrated Battle of the Bulge. But only half way – there is more to come, as we shall see: enjoyable general exercise.

5 ENJOY YOUR EXERCISE

'Firm up and feel great', write the exercise enthusiasts before knocking off for a break in front of the television. And the doctors are just as adamant: 'Continued use delays the ageing process. Use makes the organ – the heart, the bones, even the sexual organ,' writes Professor Morehouse from Los Angeles. Always the same story: *'Use it or lose it'*.

The consultant medical adviser to Rolls-Royce examined a senior executive one day and asked: 'What do *you* do for exercise?' The reply was most astonishing: 'I break concrete.'

Breaking lumps of concrete with a 10 pound sledge hammer at the bottom of your garden may be a very satisfying form of exercise. No doubt it brings beads of perspiration to the forehead and raises the respiration rate. It may, moreover, provide the means of relieving pent-up nervous tension. And so psychologically as well as physically it has merit. But it is not a very practical form of exercise to recommend for everyone.

What is needed is an enjoyable session of exercise two or three times a week for your heart, lungs and general circulatory system. But note, the key word is enjoyable. If it is not enjoyable you are not likely to persevere with it and, the more enjoyable it is the more benefit you are likely to derive from it.

Let me tell you a story told by the BBC medical correspondent in the programme 'Medicine now – what alternative,' January 1958. Mr Norman Cousins was very ill, and was given two months to live. He was in an American intensive care unit suffering from a life-threatening disease, surrounded by bottles giving him constant drip-feed when he suddenly came to a decision: 'This is no way to spend the last two months of my life.'

So he discharged himself from hospital, which was costing him an incredible amount of money, and went across the road to a first class hotel where he booked himself a room and then asked room service to bring him all the funniest films that had been made in the last 30 years;

Abbott and Costello, the Marx brothers, the lot. 'Because if I'm going to die I'm going to die laughing.'

He put the films on and he laughed and he laughed and he laughed. 'Within five days he was completely cured,' said Dr Pietroni. Medical specialists then carried out a series of tests. They were amazed at his recovery. 'Here is anecdotal evidence with a message,' said Dr Pietroni, 'a message that the power of the emotions does have a positive effect on your health and fitness.'

Enjoyment is particularly important when applied to exercise schedules. Even Olympic coaches recognise this. Gone today are the rigorously boring routines and regimentation that put so many restrictions on athletes under training. Rules, for example, that prevented an athlete from taking his wife with him on the pre-match preparation or that barred him from an occasional glass of wine. No two individuals are alike and therefore training programmes must be planned to cater for personal likes and dislikes.

We don't have to punish the body with gruelling routines for everyday fitness. There is no need to sweat to a state of near-exhaustion. It is self-defeating to grit your teeth and haul your way relentlessly through a ritual that becomes a burden to you. It only means that sooner or later you are bound to give it up.

Enjoyable exercise is the maxim of the new breed of fitness enthusiasts who have learnt to make beneficial physical activity an enjoyable part of their daily lives. They follow a balanced programme of exercise that caters for the three main aspects of fitness – sometimes called the 'S' factors – stamina, suppleness and strength. Enjoyable exercise becomes a lifetime's habit. It works.

Choose your own enjoyable exercise programme

What you are after, if you have read so far in the book, is quite clear. You want a more youthful appearance and the strength, stamina and suppleness to go with it. It has probably taken you a few years to realise that you are not quite as young as you used to be. Now you are about to start a programme that will make you look and feel better immediately. Gradually after that, we are going to build onto that programme. If you want a crash programme then you have the wrong book. Crash programmes, like all fads, inevitably fail. How many of you have tried the trendy work-outs of modern big name gurus and failed to stay the course? Come to that, how many of the big name gurus actually follow their own courses? Far better to choose a programme yourself. After all, it's your body, and you are responsible for it.

But before you select your programme keep in mind what you are after: an enjoyable session of exercise that sets in motion all the other systems of the body — those needed for repair and rejuvenation — which require that your physical activity should make you breathe more deeply and your heart beat faster.

By exercising 15 minutes a day, two or three times a week, you improve the blood supply to the heart due to the opening up of an increasing number of capillaries feeding the heart muscle. Consequently this muscle grows stronger and can pump more blood round the body with fewer and more powerful contractions.

The benefit of having a stronger heart beat is that not only do you have greater reserves to call upon from the heart itself but also that all the other systems of the body become more efficient from the infusion of life-giving oxygen: increased demands upon the lungs force them to work more efficiently in pushing more oxygen into the blood. The digestive system benefits too; fit people seem able to extract more of the essential nutrients from food and are able to expel some of the less desirable properties such as cholesterol.

But we have got to be realistic about exercise. It can be boring if it is no more than a series of basic exercises. So, if you feel this way about a specific exercise routine then forget it — for now. Get started on the more pleasurable activities — the 'play-way' to fitness outlined in the next chapter. Later you might feel more inclined to tackle a systematic conditioning programme. Meanwhile have a go at something new. It doesn't matter whether it is disco dancing or digging in the allotment. Getting started is the vital step.

For those of you who feel ready for the Basic Five Exercise Circuit, turn to pages 128 to 133 Appendix I. You will see that the exercises can be modified to suit any age and physical condition.

Be kind to yourself

Go easy to start with. Build up to a more strenuous programme gradually. You can expect to have a rosy glow and be somewhat breathless immediately after the exercise — this is an indication that you are having the right response from the heart and lungs. If you remain flushed and breathless for a long time afterwards or if you are in any way concerned about the effects of the exercise, then seek medical advice.

Consult your doctor before starting an exercise programme if you have ever had high blood pressure or heart disease, severe chest trouble such as bronchitis, severe arthritic pains in joints or back and if you are just recovering from an operation. It cannot be emphasised too much that progression should be gradual in the severity of the demands of the exercise upon your heart and lungs.

A special warning for joggers

An inquiry into the deaths of 30 experienced joggers – those who covered many miles weekly over several years – revealed that 19 died whilst out running and 6 suddenly after the exercise. 2 were found dead in bed. Three-quarters of the victims suffered from coronary heart disease. Exercise wisely. Enjoy yourself.

Dr Roger Bannister, the world's first 4-minute miler, put the whole business of exercise quite plainly, saying: 'We need a national policy that associates good health with positive enjoyment, by providing an increased network of sporting facilities of all sorts for all sections of the community.'

There are plenty of pleasurable activites to choose from. But don't be tempted into vigorous competitive games until you are really fit. It's all too easy to try and prove there's life in the old dog yet, but it can be dangerous. Obviously your exercise has got to raise the level of your respiration and heart rate for it to have a beneficial effect but take care not to overdo it in the early days. It's a question of building up stamina and developing muscles.

The old attitude to exercise was to specialise; to work at specific areas to whittle away inches or build up curves. But now exercise is more concerned with general fitness geared to give you a boost both physically and mentally.

Exercise must be a joy. There is a 'play-way' to fitness for everyday life. More opportunities are available for whatever activity you wish to choose. Fit more than one into your programme and avoid the possibility of monotony and subsequent boredom. Don't be housebound; it leads to sitting around. Get out and get active! Play your way to a younger and fitter shape.

To summarise

1) Exercise *can* be enjoyable if you choose what you want to do.
2) The most important exercise is one which makes the heart and lungs work harder. It can still be just as enjoyable as a sport.
3) If you don't enjoy your exercise you are likely to give up.
4) You don't have to push yourself until it hurts.
5) Remember you are getting fit for life − to enjoy it − not to be a world-beating athlete.
6) Look for the 'play-way' to fitness, with plenty of variety in the activity programme.

6 VARIETY IS THE SPICE OF LIFE – WITH EXERCISE

How does pop star Cliff Richard manage to look so good in his 40s? He has been topping the stressful world of show business for over 20 years. It might easily have aged him beyond recognition. Yet he could still pass for 34. What is his secret for staying young? In his own words, a commonsense approach to health.

He takes care with his meals – avoids fattening foods, cuts down on Calories and makes sure he gets his full quota of vitamins. He takes exercise through hard work and a variety of other enjoyable ways, and this, it seems, is the simple reason for him looking as young and fit as he did in the 1960s. He is not alone in this 'commonsense' approach to health. It is, in the end, the only successful one.

Mix your work, and your physical exercise and your enjoyment in a variety of ways; ideally play your way fit. For example, Kate, a 35-year-old London secretary who travels to work by underground every day, told me how she tackled the exercise business.

'Every morning, of the 60 people who get off the train at my station, about 8 of us walk up the steps – 100 of them – instead of taking the lift. It's quieter, we aren't herded together with people coughing germs all over us and we have the satisfaction of having taken some exercise at the beginning of each day. I manage a lunchtime swim once or twice a week and on Tuesday night I go ballroom dancing. At the weekend I like to get out into the country for a nice long walk and a breath of fresh air.' She is bursting with vitality. Exercise is no chore. She is playing her way to fitness. It's a regular programme and it gives her a lot of enjoyment. Even the stair walking in its own way, through a sense of satisfaction. She looks good. She feels good. And the guy in her life loves her all the more.

Stair climbing is in fact very good exercise. Five minutes of it every day is quite enough to keep your heart and lungs toned up. When you come to think of it, you can see why. It is a very vigorous exercise because the leg muscles have to lift the entire body weight 8 inches with each step forward. It takes about the same amount of energy to walk 50 yards on the level as it does to climb a flight of stairs in the average home. This surely is the cheapest and most concentrated way of taking exercise you could find. Try 10 times up and down your stairs and see if you can hold a normal conversation afterwards without too much huffing and puffing.

Moreover, did you know you could climb the height of Everest, the world's highest mountain, in 16 weeks if you walked up and down the average house staircase 30 times a day? Take out your calculator. There are usually 13 steps each 8 inches high. Multiply this by 30, divide by 12 and you'll see how you can climb 260 feet a day. Everest is 29,000 feet high – give or take a few feet – and so in 15.9 weeks to be exact at 260 feet a day you have reached the height of the summit. What an achievement and for so little time. 10 'ups and downs' takes between two to three minutes. A session of 10 in the morning, 10 at teatime and 10 later will give you all the aerobic exercise you need. Increase it to 50 a day and you'd be up Everest in nine and a half weeks! Set yourself a target. Enjoy it.

It is not quite so easy to work out the energy expenditure in all the physical recreational activities available to you but a glance at the scorecard below will give you a good guide for making your choice. Each one is graded on a 10-point scale in terms of strength, stamina and suppleness as well as showing the approximate number of Calories burnt by someone participating at an average level of play for each half hour.

'On your bike': Cycling

'Women are catching on to the idea that cycling is fun, healthy and altogether desirable for a host of reasons,' said the Sales Director of the leading cycle manufacturer, Raleigh. 'Women's cycles are the boom segment of the industry.'

Cycling is a quick way of taking exercise that tones up the whole body and burns off excess fat at the rate of 700 Calories an hour! The heart, lungs and circulatory system have to work hard but without any strain being thrown upon joints as jogging does on the knee, ankle and hip joints of the not-so-young. The smooth rhythmic movement of pedalling is especially beneficial to those with painful joints which make even walking difficult. The cycle bears the weight, the muscles provide the power.

10-POINT RATING SCALE FOR
PHYSICAL RECREATIONAL ACTIVITIES

Activity	Stamina	Suppleness	Strength	Calorie consumption per half hour
Archery	5	5	8	100
Badminton	6	8	5	185
Baseball	7	6	7	150
Basketball	8	8	6	220
Canoeing	10	6	10	420
Chopping logs	8	4	7	200
Climbing	8	6	8	280
Cricket	5	5	5	120
Cycling	10	7	8	350
Dancing (ballroom)	5	7	3	175
Dancing (disco)	7	8	3	220
Digging (garden)	7	6	6	200
Fencing	6	7	4	160
Football	8	7	8	250
Golf	4	5	6	125
Gymnastics	6	8	8	220
Ice-skating	7	8	6	200
Jogging	8	6	6	300
Judo/Karate	7	6	7	200
Rowing	10	6	10	420
Sailing	5	4	5	180
Skiing	8	6	7	240
Skipping	10	8	6	400
Squash	8	8	6	300
Swimming (hard)	8	8	7	250
Stair climbing	8	6	6	240
Tennis	6	8	6	200
Walking briskly	7	5	6	200
Weight training	8	5	10	300
Volleyball	7	7	6	210
Yoga	3	9	3	125

One of the bonuses of cycling is that you can keep fit in cycling to work. 'Why take up precious time going to a gym for aerobics when I can exercise my heart and legs with the exhilaration of sailing smoothly along at a pace that makes me pant as little or as much as I feel like?' said a lawyer friend who sits at a desk all day. The exhilaration he mentioned is indeed a positive benefit peculiar to cycling and not to be discounted lightly. It might surprise you to know that mental hospitals have used it as a treatment for people suffering from slight depression and found it to be far more effective than pills.

Remember then, that cycling should be enjoyable and not a painful chore. There are no prizes for forcing yourself up a hill when it would be easier, and safer, to get off and walk. As you make progress in your cycling, take longer rides at the weekend and shorter ones on weekdays – perhaps at a steadily increasing pace so that you cover more distance in the same time. All things considered, no other form of exercise is quite as versatile as cycling, one of the fastest growing of all sports and leisure activities today.

Squash: a game for gladiators

Squash is a gladiatorial game. Anyone who has played the game for a number of years will tell you how difficult it is not to 'take on' a younger player in the belief that guile and experience will overcome the abundant energy of youth. It is no use thinking that you will be more sensible than to fall into that trap; too many level-headed men have died on the squash court for the risks to be taken lightly.

There is no real comparison with tennis. There the risks are much smaller, for tennis is played on an open court leaving a much smaller margin for error. In a closed squash court the rallies can be very fast, furious, packed with desperate stretches done in a high temperature and with a very high pulse rate. It is not a game where you can easily coast along at your own pace, even when playing with someone of your own age group and ability. Safer to take up a less demanding activity that you can continue into later life, such as swimming.

Swimming – the ideal exercise?

Swimming is often recommended as an exercise to develop every muscle of the body in a harmonious way and this includes your heart muscle. It is of tremendous value for those who are incapacitated through injuries or nerve damage, for the body's weight is partially supported by water thus sparing sensitive joints and weakened muscles from the jarring that jogging can give. Clearly here is an activity that can provide a good deal of enjoyment and a psychological boost to those people with restricted mobility because of disabling conditions of arthritis. When painful joints are supported in water a degree of flexibility returns which is not normally seen in other situations.

Swimming is strongly recommended for restoring muscle tone after pregnancy – it strengthens particularly the back and abdominal muscles which have become stretched in childbirth. A cardiologist recently spoke about the way swimming was helping sufferers from varicose veins. The gentle but strong rhythmic movement of leg muscles acts upon the weak valves and walls of the veins like natural massage thus moving the blood along and so helping to avoid swollen veins and valves.

Are there no risks at all attached to swimming? Very few. And you can forget some of the old wives' tales about cramp due to swimming after eating a meal. According to Professor Laurence E. Morehouse, professor of Exercise Physiology at the University of California, Los Angeles, there is no scientific evidence for this myth. Cramps have never caused drowning. People will argue that food in the stomach will draw blood away from the active muscles and into the digestive tract, thus throwing a strain upon the heart working excessively hard to send oxygenated blood to the working muscles. The fact is that once energetic exercise begins the circulation of blood to the intestine is closed down, blood is sent directly to the peripheral muscles and skin. The worst that might happen through swimming soon after a heavy meal is a feeling of nausea or stitch. Ideally then you should plan your swimming so that you don't have a lot of food inside. Nor should you have a completely empty feeling.

Go to it! And think how good you'll look in that new swimsuit on the beach at Cannes, Corfu or California!

Walking is wonderful

A new US joke is that in the future Man will be born with wheels instead of feet. And it's true that most of us could walk more than we do; we could walk more briskly more often, and for longer. And then, as simply as that, we could develop a lasting habit of exercise that really is beneficial.

Leave the car parked further away from the bus stop, station or shops. Walk that extra bit. See how much extra mileage on foot you can clock up each week. Use stairs instead of lifts whenever you can; you're giving your heart and legs a bonus of healthy exercise that you would not normally have had. When you consider that two-thirds of the body's muscle mass is in the legs then it is easy to see how important it is for these muscles to be used. Otherwise they waste.

New research emphasises the therapeutic value of walking and shows how you can burn away a surprising number of unwanted Calories in this way. For example, a brisk 15 minute walk at 4 mph in the morning and the same in the evening would expend 150 Calories (5 Calories per minute). We need, for general fitness, to expend 300 Calories in physical activity each day, says Professor Morehouse, of the University of California, and this can be done in a variety of ways. Walking is one of the easiest; the balance could be made up with other enjoyable physical activities, such as tennis or dancing.

Dr Paul Dudley White, an American heart specialist, wrote: 'It has been said that a five mile walk will do more good to an unhappy but healthy adult than all the medicine and psychology in the world.' With the habit of walking well established you will feel fitter and want to take part in other rejuvenating physical activities. Nothing succeeds like success.

Walking puts weight upon your bones whilst the muscle mass is being exercised and the body reacts to this weight-bearing exercise by putting more calcium into the bone structure making it stronger and less liable to fracture, especially later in life when falls can be more serious.

Carry on dancing

It's fun, it's energetic, and it's friendly. All kinds of dancing give you good exercise. It develops co-ordination of movement, flexibility and can provide first class aerobic exercise. Beware though of taking on a long and strenuous disco session and not dropping out when you feel ready for a rest simply because you don't want to seem puffed before your partner.

Naturally, if you have not been dancing for years there will be a certain hesitancy and possible shyness about starting again. But once you have made the first move you will want to go again. Do not be put off if the first occasion is not a huge success – try again, for people who go dancing are usually friendly folk. With ballroom dancing especially you can begin at any age and there is usually a range of dances to choose from. Why not give it a try? Go on! Enjoy yourself.

Whichever activity you choose for your exercise programme remember that healthy fatigue is far better than sheer exhaustion. It's all very well to be inspired to great efforts but if you do too much at first you can do more harm than good. Take it steadily and you will soon be experiencing the exhilaration that comes from regular physical exercise. Your step will be lighter as you regain the vitality of younger days.

It could be just at this time you feel ready to have a go at a more systematic form of fitness training. One that is purposeful, bringing measurable progress in a shorter time: circuit training. Take a look at what it involves.

To summarise

1) Commonsense attitudes to exercise and diet bring the rewards you want.
2) The easiest, most effective and most readily available form of exercise is climbing up your own house stairs. Five minutes of it every day will keep you fit.
3) Take up a sport you can enjoy with a friend. You can keep each other going better in this way.
4) Embrace a variety of activities into your fitness programme. It will ensure all-round fitness.
5) When you feel fitter you might feel like more of a challenge. Why not try circuit training?

7 SHORT CIRCUIT TO FITNESS

'Does your work keep you too occupied to do anything about your fitness? Do you find sports and jogging too strenuous and time consuming? Then read about a new method . . .' Such are the opening lines of an advertisement for a piece of fitness training equipment. The words echo the thoughts of many men and women today who are looking for a quick and easy way to improve their figure and fitness.

Time, though, is precious. No one wants to waste it on futile arm waving exercises nor in travelling to sports clubs if an alternative and effective method of getting really fit is available. But how are we to choose between the countless methods presented on television, in magazines and in newspapers? We need a method that has been tried and tested. One that has withstood the fickle whims of fitness enthusiasts. And this leaves us with circuit training.

Circuit training is still the ideal routine for dedicated men and women who want to get fit quickly. And this means about 10 or 15 minutes three times a week.

What is circuit training?

As the name implies, it involves going round a circuit or series of exercises one after the other. You do a set number of repetitions of each one until you come to the first exercise again and then, if you are feeling fit enough, you do a second lap.

The task, or set number of repetitions for each exercise, is decided by a test, when you first start training, at which you try to repeat the exercise as many times as possible before fatigue makes you falter. This is the time to stop and record your score. The task for each exercise session is then set at half the maximum repetitions achieved, and, ideally, two laps of the circuit should be done at this rate. But there is nothing to be lost in starting gradually and only doing one lap for the first week. For those who are already fairly fit the task can be set at two-thirds of maximum performance and three laps completed.

51

But always start at well below your assessed capabilities. If you begin training at a comfortable rate you will attain your true level soon enough — mark the date and count the days.

What makes circuit training so popular is that you are able to see how much progress you are making in terms of strength and endurance at your next testing session. It is convincing proof that the training time has been well spent. Adjust this training task about every two weeks.

For those who wish to read more details of this method of training, the book, *Circuit Training* by Morgan and Adamson, is strongly recommended.

Training circuits

The circuits shown on pages 128 and 129, Appendix I, are designed to allow men and women of varying ability to start training at a safe level of exertion and to progress to harder work as soon as they are fit enough to do so.

When two laps of the circuit can be completed comfortably, new exercises should be introduced one at a time. Those that can be done more than 30 times maximum at the two week test should be replaced by the corresponding exercise from the next schedule. If only one new exercise is brought in at one session then no one need worry whether he or she is overtaxing strength or stamina.

The order of the exercises is arranged so that different parts of the body are exercised in rotation. The major muscle groups have in this way a little time to recover before being worked again. Keep to the order shown for both testing and training.

Circuit training can be very strenuous. You may want to start with some of the more difficult exercises. And you might be able to cope with a tough schedule, but try to avoid this temptation. Take it easy and warm up well before starting the circuit. Figure 6 shows six simple warming up exercises which can be done freely in a relaxed manner.

Before you start

Be businesslike. Check your daily routine and decide which is the most convenient time for you to exercise. Success depends on keeping to a regular routine and working enthusiastically.

The exercise will make you sweat profusely so you will need a good

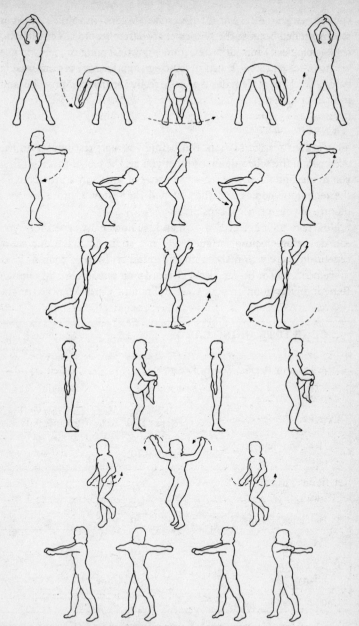

Fig. 6 Circuit training warming-up exercises

53

sponge down afterwards. Exercise before breakfast is not recommended because the sudden change from rest to violent activity is physiologically unsound and, from a practical point of view, no one wants to travel to work still perspiring slightly. An evening session twice a week (or three times if you are really keen) would probably suit most people best.

The first training session

This is your testing session. But before you start testing, try all the exercises in the schedule first so that you get the feel of them. At first you might find the movements awkward but with only a little practice the technique comes and the test will then show a more accurate picture of your physical capacity.

Now take each exercise in turn and see how many repetitions you can do before feeling fatigued. Do not strain to make one more repetition merely to make a 'round' number. Stop as soon as your movements flag or become jerky. Record your score in the 'Maximum Repetitions' column on your Circuit Training Card. You can use the

CIRCUIT TRAINING CARD						Schedule One
Date Training Begins: Weight Record						Date: Weight kgs
Exercises	Max. Reps	Trg. Task	Max. Reps	Trg. Task	Max. Reps	Trg. Task
1. Head and shoulder raising	20	10				
2. Trunk raising backwards	22	11				
3. Half knee bending	40	20				
4. Press away	28	14				
5. Stair stepping flight of 13	12	6				
Dates of Testing	.../.../...		.../.../...		.../.../...	

Further Circuits for you to tackle are given in Appendix I.

blank card or prepare your own if you don't want to deface the book. In the next column, marked 'Training Task', put in the figure that is half your maximum score. Your card will then look something like the one set out opposite.

You are now ready to start your short circuit to fitness. Attempt one lap at your training task for each exercise, and if you still feel capable then attempt two. But be ready to rest at any time. (Details and drawings in pages 28 to 133, Appendix I.) You must go slowly at first.

Making progress

1) Do not push yourself too hard in the first week.
2) Test yourself after two weeks and record the maximum scores.
3) Replace the exercise if you can do it more than 30 times with one from the corresponding part of the next schedule.
4) Gradually introduce new exercises until you have reached Schedule Three.
5) If you are feeling capable of harder work at this stage, increase the task to two thirds of maximum performance at each exercise.

You are now taking responsibility for your own life, for what you eat and for what you give your body. No faddism – no fancy diets, no fast way to new health, no fake cure-alls, but a realistic down-to-earth course of diet plus exercise for the average mid-lifer.

But there is more to staying young longer and keeping fit than physical activity and diet. You have to learn how to deal with the psychological side, the emotional aspect of health and fitness. And this is particularly true when it comes to sexual fitness, which deserves a chapter for itself.

To summarise

1) Circuit training has proved itself over many years.
2) It exercises all the major muscle groups and develops efficiency of the heart and lungs.
3) You need no equipment.
4) You can progress at your own pace.
5) Progress can be seen and measured.

8   SEXUAL FITNESS

Sally Penfold was an attractive, outgoing woman of 37 when she first became aware that her sex life was not just boring but almost moribund. She had been married for 17 years and had two teenagers at home studying for exams.

'I suppose, like many other couples of our age, we'd had a normal rather mundane sort of sex life without much novelty or variation, believing that certain methods of love-making were right and proper and that to try anything else would be degrading. Well, all that led to was boredom. We had sex less and less frequently. Something had to be done. For one reason I felt I was wanting sex more than I used to yet my husband seemed to have lost interest. So I got a book out of the library and began to jolt him out of his rut. I brought a bit of surprise into our bedtime. And it worked.' A wise move.

Sally's situation is not unusual. Men and women in their late 30s are often preoccupied with other aspects of their lives than sex; they are so busy with their careers, earning money, paying off the mortgage, being housewives, mothers, and fathers, that they lose sight of sex. And they don't bother much. Furthermore, having teenage children in the house doesn't help much. Parents sometimes feel embarrassed about making love in bed at night with only a thin partitioning wall of the modern house between bedrooms. But why should they be embarrassed? Would it not be more natural to let their children know that sex did go on in mid-life and later as a physical expression of love? It would create a healthy atmosphere, surely, for children to grow in. There is no reason why the parents' sex life should deteriorate simply because teenage and younger adults are about the house. Parents who are at ease with their own sexuality will no doubt help their children to feel at ease with theirs.

Now, back to Sally. Part of her problem was boredom. She realised that it was never too late – or too early – to open new doors to romance. She did well to seek more knowledge – there are plenty of good books on the subject. Two books spring to mind – *Enjoy Sex in the Middle Years* by Dr Christine Sandford, and the well known *Joy of Sex* by Dr Alex Comfort.

Knowledge, reliable and trustworthy, as opposed to hearsay and old wives' tales, can often be the simple answer to many of the problems that bedevil marital bliss. People grow up with such a mass of myths and misconceptions about sex that it is small wonder that when, in later life, changes occur they fail to cope with them properly. Feelings of inadequacy, resentment, and rejection grow, get mixed together and are then suppressed, only to emerge again in angry asides and taunts during arguments on other matters.

It is right that people should seek to solve sexual problems. They have a great effect on health and marriage. Today, most of us know about sexual hang-ups and the resultant emotional problems – on paper. But do we really know what is going on in our partner's mind?

You have only to look at the recent surveys. The agony aunt of an American magazine wrote in her column: 'Tell me about your sex life.' A staggering 64,000 women replied. More recently *Woman* magazine did a survey of the nation's sex life and 15,000 readers took part. They sent in detailed reports of their love and sexual experiences; the frequency of love-making and the fantasies involved. Then, of course, there are the earlier celebrated surveys of Kinsey and the one by Masters and Johnson.

From all these what emerges is an increasing willingness of women and men – particularly those of the 39-year-old vintage – to talk about their problems freely. And what also becomes abundantly clear is that the joys of sex and love are not the exclusive privileges of youth. Men and women can go on enjoying a fully satisfying and active sex life until the end of their days.

They *can* go on – but do they? Unfortunately many do not. For a variety of reasons. You have only to look at the letters to counsellors of the problem page of women's magazines to see what can and does happen. And at 40, not 60. Here is a typical letter: 'I'm in my early 40s, married for nearly 20 years and we have two children, 15 and 12. Our sex life has never been satisfactory – my husband has never been particularly interested although I have tried to change him. Gradually our sex life has become almost non-existent. And when I tried to talk to him about it saying it was for me a very necessary part of marriage, he became quite angry and said words to the effect that what on earth did a woman of my age want with sex? That there must be something wrong with me. At first I felt like finding the nearest available man, but that is no answer. Marriage Guidance would be no good as he would never agree to go. I don't know where to go for advice.'

Naturally the magazine counsellor agreed that it was nonsense to think there was an age after which we should not be interested in sex. She advised the wife to seek all help possible from the Marriage Guidance Council even if the husband refused to go. It might make him realise this was a serious matter and she might pick up some ideas about how to make her husband change his attitude.

Clearly it is not always the woman who is not interested in sex. OK – there is the threadbare joke about the wife having migraine again or being too tired for sex. But who's to blame? What stimulus has the man provided all evening slumped in his chair, thumbing through the evening paper, watching television and then making a half-hearted pass at his partner in bed? Who would be roused from lethargy by that? Where has the gallant of former days gone? Has he lost all appeal? And this is why so many women fantasise – at least 50 per cent of them from current surveys – when making love.

Valerie, 37, said: 'I suppose I fantasise by pushing aside all thoughts of myself as a wife and mother and create an image of myself as just a woman again being desired passionately by a man.'

Sometimes though, a man fears that he might not be able to express his passionate desire with the virility of former days. And there is nothing which brings about impotence more than fear of failure, for man's sexual potency depends on psychological factors more than any other bodily function. A temporary loss of desire or a temporary failure can occur at any age. In the early years, however, an occasional failure may be taken in stride. But when it occurs around the 40-year-old mark it might covince a man that 'this is it' – that he has reached the end of his sex life. Consequently when he next attempts to make love with his partner he might have doubts and fear he will not be up to it. This attitude of mind is almost bound to bring failure. Thus, after a few embarrassing trials – determined but sabotaged with doubts – which end unsuccessfully, he stops altogether. He comes to regard himself as 'over the hill', totally impotent. It is a false and foolish assumption. There is no need to fear failure. Once fear is overcome the situation improves in ways that seem miraculous.

What men and women have to recognise is the fact that certain changes in sexuality do happen in mid-life. Men do tend to take longer to get an erection, women do not always respond as they used to do. But there is no need to fear these changes. They can in fact be the gateway to new gardens of pleasure. Though a man might take longer to reach a firm erection he can usually maintain it for much longer and delay his ejaculation thereby contributing to mutual pleasure.

We should not look upon these and other changes as a fading of sexual performance. In fact the sooner the term 'performance' is forgotten the better. Sex is not a competitive activity with two partners competing against one another. When they can talk freely and genuinely want to please each other there is much to be gained.

It is like the two Chinese pictures of Heaven and Hell. In both pictures people are sitting at a table laden with good food but with 10 feet long chopsticks that are too long to carry the food from the plate to mouth. In the picture of Hell everybody is trying to solve the problem by tilting their head back, struggling with outstretched arms and spilling most of the food. But in Heaven people are happily eating away – feeding each other. There is no problem. You have to help each other.

The first step towards improving a sexual relationship is a frank talk. Of course it is never easy to be absolutely frank about personal feelings and it can be especially difficult for some people when the subject is sex. Fortunately though, inhibitions are being swept aside; the trend in society today is towards a healthier and more open discussion of what partners find exciting and pleasurable. More and more couples find that they can tackle sexual problems best as a couple. They might go together to see their own doctor who may be able to offer help immediately by explaining how sexual dysfunction comes from other causes such as smoking (see chapter 16). He might put them in touch with a psychosexual therapist. Once this rapport has been established and the problem tackled in a positive way, success is assured.

Ringing the bell

The volcano blowing its top – the male orgasm – is an intensely pleasurable experience. But what about women? Can they reach a similar peak of pleasure? They can. And they should, if sex is going to satisfy and delight both partners equally.

This is where we have to get rid of another bit of sexual bunkum. One that Sally mentioned earlier – the common misconception – a relic from Victorian prudery perhaps – that the only acceptable form of sex is for the man to put his penis into a vagina and pump away until he falls off exhausted from his own orgasm. Nonsense! Few women can reach orgasm this way.

Several studies carried out over the last few years indicate that – contrary to what's generally believed – most women do not reach orgasm during intercourse. They reach it only during love play. Women who 'ring the bell', 'blow their fuse' or 'pop the cork', during intercourse, are the fortunate few – only a minority.

Mutual pleasure must be the aim of good sex. To think otherwise is selfish and destroys sexual harmony. Gratification for both partners, whatever their sexual problems might be, can be achieved naturally through loving cuddles, caressing and stroking leading to mutual masturbation. 'We should accept masturbation as a "healthy means of sexual expression",' writes Elizabeth Stanley, specialist in Obstetrics at St. George's Hospital, London.

Good sex – good health

That sexual fitness and satisfaction are closely connected with general wellbeing is generally agreed. Good sex is biologically desirable, say specialists in many fields who have found that disabilities often stem from an unsatisfactory sex life. Men and women around the 40-year-old mark are particularly vulnerable.

Take for example men and women who suffer pain down the neck and arm, 'pins and needles' in their little finger, sometimes attributed to a 'trapped nerve', and have to wear a surgical collar as a splint. The pain is real, often excruciating and notoriously unpredictable. It comes and goes without any degenerative changes in the vertebrae showing on X-ray plates. Suddenly, though, the pain may go and the symptoms disappear. The cure? Often this 'miraculous' relief follows a congenial marriage or a robust love affair. And the collar is never worn again.

Sexual dysfunction, fear of impotency, can make life a misery for men and women. It can lead to loss of confidence, anxiety, loss of ambition, depression, alcoholism and the chronic ill-health that is likely to go with all these conditions. Sexual incompatibility is a major cause of marriages breaking up – especially in the divorce-prone age of 39 plus. And, it is not surprising if, after such a traumatic experience, there comes another phase of emotional difficulties, further anxiety, deeper depression and sickness.

There is no need for much of this misery. Everyone owes it to themselves and their partners to seek happiness through sexual fulfilment and the way to achieve this is through a down-to-earth approach sweeping away all the inhibitions about frank discussion of problems. They will not be solved through the patent aphrodisiac remedies, once hidden discreetly under the counter but now socially acceptable and one of the best selling products of the pharmaceutical industry. The best they can give anyone is hope and faith and by the 'placebo' effect restore sexual function. Now forget the aphrodisiacs, forget the failures and forget your own needs. Concentrate hard on pleasing your partner. Go forward with confidence and the problem will disappear like morning mist as if it had never been there. And you are back with the old equation: Good Sex = Good Health = Good Relationship.

To summarise

1) Talk frankly about sex, and any problems you have, with your partner.
2) Think more about giving pleasure than taking.
3) Cuddles and caresses can bring wonderful rewards.
4) Cure your sexual hang-ups and you can cure the pain in your neck, the ache in your back and remove a possible cause of emotional stress.

9 HOW TO REPLACE STRESS WITH SERENITY

Late one Sunday afternoon last summer Jennifer Henderson decided to quit her job. She was one of three doctors in a village practice on the outskirts of York, England.

It happened quite suddenly. So suddenly in fact that she didn't realise she had made up her mind until she told her husband half an hour later over tea. That was last August. Now, six months later, she is a different woman; inwardly content and enthusiastic about her new job as an occupational medicine consultant with a state industry. What actually happened?

Her words went something like this: 'I suppose it was the last straw that broke the camel's back. I was weeding the border at the bottom of my garden, a job I've been putting off for weeks, when I heard shouting coming from the house. Voices raised in argument. One of them was my husband's. Then a red faced, heavily built man of about 40 came storming through the patio door onto the lawn shouting as he approached me "She's got to come, it's her job, I have a right".

'I walked towards him, trailing my spade. "Doctor, you've got to come, it's urgent".

' "What's the matter?" I said.

' "Well, on Friday we had a new electric cooker delivered. It didn't work so we went back to the showroom and kicked up such a fuss they came and fitted a new one. Now that one doesn't work. We've got friends coming to dinner and my wife's in hysterics, sitting in the middle of the kitchen floor chucking plates and cups and smashing everything in sight."

' "I don't know anything about electric cookers," I said. But I drove to the hysterical wife's house and found her sweeping up the broken crockery.

'I came home, threw myself into an armchair and sipped my tea. It was then that the words came out. "I'm packing it in. I'd rather be on the dole than harassed like this. Not a minute to call my own".'

Do you ever get the feeling that your life is out of control? That you have so much to do you don't quite know where to start and so much to remember that something is bound to be forgotten? If so, you are under stress.

Yet there are people who are taking everything in their stride without apparent anger, worry, fear or frustration. They seem to go through life unperturbed and comparatively free from sickness or depression, enjoying life to the full. And it shows in their face as vivacity, one of the attractive features of being young. The worriers look old before their time. Anxiety lines the face and plays havoc with health.

What is stress?

Stress is a prolonged emotional tension that produces real changes in the body chemistry and structure of quite normal people. And it seems to come to people more in the late 30s and early 40s than at any other time. It is a time when things go wrong and marriages break up. We have to guard against this stress and replace it with serenity. It's a mental attitude we have to tackle.

Everyone knows that certain thoughts bring an automatic response beyond your control; shame makes you blush, fear quickens your heart beat, and sexual desire arouses organs for function. Think of savoury food when you are hungry and you salivate. There are many such examples of how mind and body react closely to a situation. Take for example the case of Meg.

She was a woman who felt insecure in her job, constantly being criticised. One Friday evening after an unpleasant row with her boss, she left work to spend a weekend away from it all with friends. It was a pleasant break indeed. But when she was approaching home on her return journey she suddenly broke into a rash which covered her whole body. For weeks it stayed that way. Then she found another job and the rash never returned. The cause was obvious.

Pent up emotions and stress express themselves through various parts of the body; symptoms might appear merely as a rash, shortness of breath or a pounding heart. But in other cases, actual organic disorders can develop. Hypertension, thyroid malfunction, asthma, skin eruptions, ulcers, some cancers, and coronary thrombosis are often attributed to stress.

Not all stress, however is harmful. Simple, occasional stress may indeed be beneficial – a challenge that adds spice to life, but continuous and excessive tension is ageing. It damages the body and tell-tale signs appear. Tensed muscles remain cramped, blood pressure stays too high, interest in food wanes and with increasing frequency come unreasonable flashes of anger. Sleep is difficult and chronic fatigue makes life a misery. Gradually your physical condition deteriorates, there is a lack of interest in sex, sometimes loss of weight, and ultimately psychosomatic sickness which may take one of a wide variety of forms.

Occasionally such illnesses are labelled as 'psychosomatic' in a sneering sort of way, as if the sickness were simply in the mind, imaginary. But this is far from the truth. Psychosomatic illnesses have symptoms that look just as alarming on X-ray plates and electrocardiograms as organically caused ones do. It is an accepted medical fact that your mind can make you ill, make you older or keep you young.

Mark, 44, gave up his job in a school where he was Head of a Languages Department because he recognised the warning signs. 'You're taking a big risk at your age, giving up a job,' his friends told him. 'Not so much of a risk as the one I'd be taking if I stayed with that mob of hooligans and self-seeking Head wanting a medal from Other Beggars' Efforts,' he would reply. Now he is a different man, happier and healthier, working for the Forestry Commission – for less money and far less stress. It is a safe bet that he will be drawing his pension longer than the colleagues he left behind.

The message is clear – 'Ease up. You have no need to kill yourself'.

Who is likely to suffer from stress?

Stress is a common complaint. Many are afflicted without realising it for the deterioration in health develops slowly. Therefore we must be on our guard and learn how to release pent up pressure of nervous tension that has gradually built up. Prevention is better than cure.

Barricades can be built to protect your peace of mind; shun situations that increase tension. Learn to laugh off a dangerous argument before it even develops, walk away from people you know will 'needle' you. 'My life is in the hands of any rascal who chooses to annoy me,' said surgeon John Hunter, who had been suffering from cardiac pain. Tragically he proved himself right. After a stormy committee meeting at St. George's Hospital he died from a heart attack.

New research into stress in America reveals that a certain type of person is most likely to become a victim to stress disorders, especially coronaries. They are people of type 'A' behaviour which makes them forever in a state of urgency, competitiveness and easily aroused hostility. Surprisingly, few of us escape this label. Dr. Meyer Friedman, Director of Recurrent Coronary Prevention project in San Francisco, said 75 per cent of the adult population display varying degrees of type 'A' behaviour.

The characteristics of this type 'A' behaviour are seen in someone who often tries to do two things at once, walks fast, leaves the table quickly after finishing a meal, makes a fetish of being on time and never seems able to sit down and do nothing.

Few of us would like to admit that we are possible candidates for nervous disorders and consequently we tend to attribute the physical symptoms of sickness to physical causes. For example, because men who suffer from ulcers are put on a light diet we are inclined to assume that food has caused the trouble. Yet this is rarely the case. Frustration, fear, anger, and anxiety cause more ulcers, duodenal, gastric, and in the colon, than do fatty foods. The duodenal ulcer sufferer is usually the ambitious man bound up with the worries of his work. When the pressure of responsibility increases he worries about his ability to cope and his ulcer gets worse with the increasing nervous tension. In dire cases of excessive worry, the man may go down with a haemorrhage or perforation. Remove the worry, relax the tension, and the ulcer usually heals.

Relieving the tension

On the sharp corners of motor racing tracks there is often an escape road for the driver who approaches too fast and realises at the last moment that he just cannot take the bend. He then drives safely off the course instead of risking a serious accident from attempting the impossible.

High-pressure living can be compared with high-speed motor racing. There comes a time when risks must be accurately assessed and appropriate action taken. Those who feel they cannot make it must take an escape route for a day, get away from the rush, the jangling telephones and worry. Do as the late General Sir Brian Horrocks recommends in his book, *A Full Life:* take the private lane to another world which every man who lives a hectic well-filled life must have. For some the lane might lead to a flower garden, a vegetable plot, workshop or shelves of books. The General's lane led down to the water's edge where a small boat lay at its moorings.

Tranquillisers

Your doctor might prescribe tranquillisers of the Valium®, Ativan®, Mogadon®, and Dalmane® group as a short-term measure for relieving intense anxiety. They can get you over a crisis when stress could be too much of a handicap amidst a mass of other worrisome tasks to be done; as for example with business collapse, bereavement or divorce. But many doctors now are cautious about prescribing these drugs over a longer period than three or four months. There are not only side effects to be considered but a real risk of dependency developing. Then, cutting down can be a problem. It has to be done with care otherwise it can lead to a number of strange sensations causing a feeling of panic. Decrease the dose slowly. As one woman who was on a high daily dose of Ativan® explained: 'I was determined to get off tranquillisers. I was only half alive but it was not easy. What I did was to knock off half a pill at midday for a week or two then half off the morning and later half off the evening over a period of three or four months until I was left with just half a pill for the evening. When that finally went I felt great. I'd really done it. I was alive again. So I celebrated with the first glass of sherry I'd had for well over a year'.

Tranquillising drugs reduce your sense of alertness. Worries and problems become more remote. But they are not solved. Eventually these problems have to be recognised. You might not be able to solve them right away but time usually does. Although there is a definite place for tranquillisers to be taken under medical supervision, there does come a time when you can say to your doctor that you feel ready to face life with all its stress without the buffer of sedation. And the earlier you make this decision the easier it will be to get off the pills, for good.

Getting rid of stress symptoms

The dash-about type 'A' people, subject to stress disorders, are advised to walk, talk and eat more slowly, play games to lose, write down things that spark anger, smile at others and laugh at yourself, do one thing at a time, admit to being wrong and stop interrupting other people.

Mr. John Vaccarello, a gas inspector, was one of Dr. Friedman's type 'A' patients who needed special counselling on ways to release tension. He twitched, sighed, answered questions without a moment's thought and said that slow drivers and long traffic jams made him mad. He suffered two heart attacks. Now, after counselling on ways to relax, he listens to music in his car, stops at amber lights rather than racing through them and observes others whilst waiting in line, imagining what their lives are like.

There are many ways of removing tension and relaxing more. Gentle rhythmic exercise, like swimming and cycling, is an effective way of getting rid of the symptoms caused by the stresses of everyday life. The mind and muscular systems relax into the rhythm and stress is eased away. Games and sports enjoyed in the open air are invigorating. They take the mind off problems and provide an outlet for pent-up pressure. Frustration and tension can, in a couple of hours, be replaced by a feeling of exuberance and wellbeing.

For senior executives and women running a home as well as a job, time to relax and think in congenial surroundings is essential. A difficult situation can often be seen more clearly from a golf course or hillside track. Problems assume their proper proportions.

Periods of quiet meditation and positive relaxation are a great help. It gives time for batteries to be recharged. Here is something we can all benefit from. Once a day, preferably in the early evening, set aside a regular period of half an hour for positive relaxation. It can prove to be like an elixir of life which refreshes and rejuvenates both mind and body.

An advertising executive I know spends his days amidst the bustle of newspaper offices and fashion houses. He goes home every evening at 5 pm and looks forward to the bliss of his relaxation routine. After a warm drink he adopts one of the postures shown in Figure 7 on p 72 and spiritually floats away from the world. In half an hour the drive of his job seeps out of his system and he is a new man.

The person who needs a regular relaxation period more than anyone is the mother of a family of small children. Even more so if she is working at another job as well. Her work seems endless, repetitive and extremely taxing. She really needs a bracer of positive relaxation. It is the only way that she can restore the energy she needs to cope cheerfully with all the chores that face her every day.

What we have to do first of all is to achieve a positive relaxation of the body. Just as the mind affects the body, so, conversely, the body affects the mind. If we relax physically our mind tends to relax too. There are various postures which prove effective in achieving the degree of physical relaxation required. They are fully explained in the next chapter.

To summarise

Six steps to serenity

1) *Count 10 before allowing any reaction to anger or frustration.* By delaying the response you automatically reduce its force. Remember that what is important is not the matter that disturbs you but how you respond.
2) *Practise mental withdrawal.* 'Every man has some art by which he steals his thoughts away from his present state' wrote Doctor Samuel Johnson. 'Many have no happier moments than those they pass in solitude, abandoned to their own imagination'. There are times when we have to pull the shutters down on all the irritating aspects of our lives and retreat into the peace and quiet of our own inner dreamworld where the sun is shining and we are doing our own thing. When President Truman was asked how he coped with the stress of his job he replied, 'I have a foxhole in my mind where no man can bother me, into which I periodically retire'. We can all have this luxury or recession from life. Daydreaming was what they called it at school. We just need to practise it more often.
3) *Take a daily walk.* Observe carefully your surroundings. It is invigorating and takes the mind off problems. *Smile deliberately whether you feel like it or not,* for it has been said by psychologists that it is almost impossible to think miserable thoughts when you turn the corners of your mouth upwards. Greet people you pass cheerfully, you will be surprised at the number of appreciative smiles you get in return.
4) *Learn a new game or a musical instrument.* Physical activity

68

outdoors gives you a pleasant feeling of fatigue which helps you to sleep; playing a musical instrument is equally relaxing and provides a sense of achievement.

5) *Take an early evening nap or go to bed early occasionally.* But do not just slump in a chair in front of the television for you wake up feeling worse than ever. Go to the quiet of your bedroom and adopt a positive relaxation posture. (See page 72.) Sleep, 'the balm of hurt minds', has been accepted for centuries as the most important healing agent of all.

6) *Learn how to side-step trouble.* It is surprising how many problems will solve themselves if you just avoid them for a little while. You know the people who are likely to upset you: avoid them.

That's it then. Come to terms with your work. Accept the annoyances and let them float by leaving you unmoved. Getting angry can be a risky business in mid-life. Once again, it's for you to make a simple choice. Are you going to choose serenity with its incalculable blessings or are you going to let ambition, anger, jealousy, fear, or a combination of emotions push you to the brink of breakdown? It's up to you. Far better to avoid such risks if you can.

10   ARE YOU TAKING A CALCULATED RISK?

In some men and women there is an impulse that makes them want to climb mountains, or to drive a car faster than anyone on earth or to be the first person on another planet. It is a spirit of adventure. There is an equally potent driving force which appears as ambition in others who want to reach the top in a profession, business or creative art.

Neither of these forces can be quenched by advice to 'take it easy'. But to the mountaineer, racing motorist or astronaut the dangers are evident, risks can be calculated and physical preparation is part of the planning for success. The ambitious must plan too. Though the risks for them are not as exciting nor as evident, they are just as real, and ignoring them does not remove them.

Most of us are ambitious. We fix our sights on a target and set out to overcome all difficulties by energetic effort, but there is a limit to the strain the body can stand. There comes a time when we must pause and take stock of our commitments, of the way we are wearing ourselves out. We know that we should balance work with play, make time for exercise and relaxation. But because time is short, 'tomorrow will do' is often the attitude adopted. Tomorrow may be too late.

When it comes to modifying our life-style we are inclined to gamble, to put off for a few days, weeks, or years the action we should take now. Sometimes it is a justifiable and calculated risk but more often it is likely to be mere procrastination, foolhardy and irresponsible. We allow ourselves to be pushed on by the pressure of events and the driving force within. We say we are too busy and have no time for relaxation and recreation. It is a short sighted policy which inevitably takes its toll.

Well then, what is the answer? It is easy to give advice and to run other people's lives yet so difficult to order our own. Nevertheless, difficult though it may be, if we accept the fact that stress is potentially harmful, then we must consider how we can best get rid of the tensions that cause it. Somehow the week has to be planned so that adequate time is set aside for positive relaxation planned with the same thoroughness as the mountaineer plans his expeditions so that the known risks can be tackled with the maximum expectancy of success. No one can now say that these risks stemming from stress have not been widely publicised and confirmed by medical authorities world-wide. It is up to each one of us to guard against them and not to rely on others. We must start now.

How can we begin? We can start by relaxing the body. Relaxation of tense muscles is strongly recommended as a positive way of dealing with stress and exhaustion. People who can relax at intervals during the day have more energy to spare, they are less irritable, less aggressive, less fatigued. Less likely to have heart attacks. But the relaxation must be more than merely slumping in a chair. It must be purposeful and positive.

Techniques of positive relaxation

Just as the mind affects the body, so, conversely the body affects the mind. If we relax physically, our minds relax too.

There is always a certain amount of tension in muscles, a form of contraction that persists to a variable degree even in rest. This contraction is most evident in the postural muscles which maintain the body upright, and the number of fibres working at any one time is governed by a reflex mechanism which operates whenever the postural muscles are stretched or the body balance disturbed. Obviously the force of gravity affects muscles more in standing than in sitting and least of all in lying. Consequently, if we are to achieve maximum relaxation of muscle tension we must lie down and support all the major segments of the body so that the muscles controlling them are not stretched. Some relaxed lying postures are described below. Choose whichever is most comfortable for your own body. They are all of roughly equal merit.

Back-lying relaxation position

A firm base is essential for relaxing in the lying position. Softly sprung beds do not give enough support. If a firmly supportive bed is not available then the floor is better with a pad of folded blankets or duvet. Lie down on your back and place a small pillow under your head to prevent it from rolling sideways. Put another pillow under the knees to hold them in a slightly flexed position so that tension is taken off the

71

hamstring muscles at the back of the legs, thus allowing the pelvis to roll backwards and the lumbar spine to rest firmly on the pad or bed. The arms should lie a little way from the body, palms upwards. Finally, the feet ought to be supported to prevent movement at the ankle joint. In this lying position no muscles are being stretched or partly tensed to hold joints.

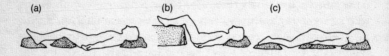

Fig. 7   Relaxed lying positions:
     (a) Back-lying relaxation position
     (b) Half-lying leg raised position
     (c) Relaxed front-lying position

Complete relaxation can now be achieved. (See Fig. 7(a).)

Half-lying leg raised position

This is a really good restful position to adopt at the end of a tiring day when your legs feel heavy with hours of standing and walking. Lie on your back with the buttocks close to the side of the bed. Flex your hips and knees at right angles and let the bed support the whole of the lower leg as shown in fig. 7(b). Knees can fall comfortably apart. Place a soft pillow under the curve of your neck. Let your arms flop, palms upwards away from the body.

In this position, accumulated waste-products of fatigue drain away from the legs, the abdomen falls flat, the small of your back rests comfortably on the floor because the tension has been taken off the hip flexor muscles attached to the spine and your chest is free for deep breathing.

Relaxed front-lying position

Lie on your front with head turned to one side and resting on a pillow. Put another pillow under the hips, abdomen and lower ribs to prevent hollowing of the back and relieve the pressure on the chest. This is particularly important for women as it avoids compression of the breasts.

72

Inducements to effective relaxation

First of all ensure that you are warm. The room should be well ventilated but not to the extent of being chilly. Loosen all tight clothing and remove belts. A warm bath is a good forerunner to a relaxation routine.

Try to put your mind at rest by repeating, chant-like, to yourself, 'breathe and let go, breathe and let go'. Allow no other thoughts to enter your head. After a few moments let your mind flit lightly over every part of your body from toes to top of the head consciously trying to induce limpness into muscles and tendons. Gradually joints and limbs will seem to sag more and more until everywhere feels pleasantly lax. By this time you might have dropped off to sleep. A wise precaution is to set an alarm or cook's timer for the period you have allowed for the relaxation. It ensures you don't have to worry about the time and keep looking at the clock.

Some people find general relaxation difficult to achieve. For them the maximal contraction method is often effective. Muscles react to forceful contraction by effecting a correspondingly greater degree of relaxation in the opposing muscle groups. For example, if you try to straighten your leg whilst a heavy weight holds it bent, the hamstring muscles will automatically relax to a greater degree the more you contract the knee extensor muscles. Consequently, using this physiological phenomenon, a comfortable degree of general relaxation can be achieved by progressively contracting and then relaxing every major muscle, group by group, from the toes upwards to the facial muscles.

This 'tense and let go' method is not new. Dr Edmund Jacobson reported successful results in the treatment of tension in the early 1930s and since then therapists trained in his methods have spread the technique throughout America and Britain. In the 60s and 70s the method was adapted slightly and is now better known as the Mitchell method of relaxation.

The way to achieve maximum results comes through practice – which you can do at any time: in the office, watching television or sitting at traffic lights in your car.

Further relaxation techniques

Now, as you are reading this page, pause and think about the muscles of your neck: are they taut or relaxed? Can you rest your head and let those muscles go limper? Yes, you can. From this easily recognised feature of muscular tension try to pick out other points in the body where stress is evident. Alter your posture to accommodate a more relaxed balance between muscle groups. One thing you must do immediately if you have been caught in this position is to uncross your legs. This piece of advice is given to all patients in the Killingbeck Heart Hospital, Leeds, which specialises in treating heart conditions. Crossing the legs is not only a position of muscular tension but it is also a dangerous way of impeding the flow of blood through the circulatory system.

Soon, by training yourself to feel tension in muscles you will be able to detect sensations of stress as they are conveyed along the afferent nerves of the body.

Here is how to start your training. Sit in a comfortable, preferably high-backed chair, rest your arms flat along the arms. Now drop your shoulders towards your feet. Make a conscious effort to pull them down. Now let go and feel the relaxed position of those muscles which had been holding the shoulders in the previous position. Next, keeping the arms on the arms of the chair, push them away from the body against the resistance of the material of the chair-arm. Relax, and this will bring a positive reciprocal relaxation in opposing muscle groups. Now it is the turn of the wrist and hand muscles. Extend your hand backwards from the wrist and push your fingers out as widely as possible. Relax and feel the new sensation of looseness in all the muscles of the forearm which control hand and wrist movement. For the large muscle groups of the legs turn the hips outwards and force your legs apart without any apparent movement of the legs or feet. Now register the new feeling throughout the upper leg muscle groups. Finally, for the feet and ankles, push your feet downwards away from the face, raising the heel. Now relax and feel the whole body in a state of complete repose.

Throughout the positive relaxation routine, breathing should be free, fairly deep and slow without being kept to an unnaturally enforced rhythm. Gradually, as the sensation of complete relaxation is appreciated, you will be able to drop into a blissfully relaxed pose as easily as a master of Yoga, and you will bless the day you learned how to do it. Why? Because the physical and mental make-up of the body are so inter-dependent that deliberate physical relaxation cannot fail to have a beneficial effect upon all systems.

To summarise

1) Help your mind to relax by seeking professional counselling in your locality. An approach to your Medical Practitioner could be the first step.
2) Use techniques of meditation and positive relaxation as a regular part of your life.
3) Get rid of pent-up emotions such as fear, anxiety, anger and jealousy – they can be as harmful to health as excessive eating, smoking and drinking.

Once you have developed the ability to relax you will find that the body's own marvellous powers of renewal and revitalisation can be working more efficiently for you.

11 THE SECRET OF
SELF-RENEWAL

'If you are reading this on 1 April you can have a silkier, smoother, younger looking skin by 10 April . . .' so ran the advertisement for cosmetic cream in one of the upmarket fashion magazines. Instant beauty. Magical rejuvenation.

Is it beyond belief? Sudden transformations are possible. We have all experienced them at times. A sudden surge of supreme well-being, filling us with so much vitality that we rub our hands with glee and feel on top of the world. Something delightful has happened. An unusual opportunity, exciting news, a challenge comes with a letter or 'phone call. It stimulates the body into a complex energy-boosting reaction. The pituitary and adrenal glands pour out secretions which instantly tone you up physically to meet the situation. Your mind has invigorated your body.

But this, you may say, is only a short-term effect. True, but mental attitudes have long-term influences too. We can, and must, ensure they are as beneficial as possible. This is the secret of self-renewal.

Scientists worldwide are recognising more than ever before that the mind can revitalise the body, and that we have therefore to harness that hidden power that lies within each one of us. It is possible and more effective than pots of patented face cream, and we are often doing it without realising what we are doing.

Look, for example, how this power of the mind can help in healing. When doctors try to discover the exact benefits of a new drug they will carry out 'double blind' tests. In these carefully monitored tests, patients in a similar stage of the same sickness are divided into groups, all appearing to take the same pill or medicine. But, in fact, only one group is being given the new drug, whilst the other group is given pills that to all intents and purposes look the same but contain no drug whatsoever – they are placebos.

Now, the strange fact emerging from these tests is that at least one third of the patients who take these 'empty' placebo pills recover like those who are receiving the real drug, provided they believe that they are in fact receiving it. And the recovery rate is even more marked if the doctor or nurse who gives the pill is an inspiring 'salesman' persuading the patient of the power the pills have to make them better.

Here we have an excellent and irrefutable example of how your mind can help your body. This being so, can we become fitter, healthier, and even younger by positive thinking or belief? Faith, we know, has a miraculous healing record. 'The power of the mind in these matters,' writes former Bishop of London, Dr Leslie Weatherhead, 'is so immense that it is hard to say what the limits are, or what cannot be achieved. If the mind accepts the suggestion that better health is returning, then in some ways that seem miraculous, it gets its orders carried out.'

All right then. We must believe in ourselves and give the body-mechanism a good chance to work well. But to do this we must first free the mind from crippling emotional hang-ups.

Control your emotions and reap the benefits

Nobody cares for the cold fish who never shows emotions. But it is one thing to be a cold fish and another to let your emotions run riot through your body wrecking your health. Somehow you have to exert control: it's your responsibility.

How do we come to grips with these emotions? What exactly are they and how do we recognise them for what they are?

At one time psychologists said that we only know when we are feeling an emotion when we see the physical symptoms working in ourselves. We know, for example, that we are embarrassed when we blush, that we are angry when we grind our teeth, breathe more deeply and clench our fists. And we know we are sad when we cry.

That was what they said. But what happens when these signs of emotional disturbance are hidden – even from yourself?

'I was absolutely livid. I've never been so angry in my life,' said Liz. 'But I kept my cool and told him that if he wanted the department run in that underhand fashion he would just have to find someone else. It was only later, as I got into my car that I realised how up-tight I was. My hands were shaking so much I couldn't get my ignition key in. God knows what would have happened if I'd driven off then. I just sat and switched on the radio until I calmed down. It was a bit frightening actually.'

Here Liz was showing that we don't always know the intensity of emotions that bubble inside us at particular times. And few people would like to admit that they are affected in this way either.

However, if we are going to give our body-power the best possible conditions in which to work for us, in repair and recuperation, then we have to do something about destructive emotions. Firstly we must recognise them and vent them. Get them out, not bottle them up. Secondly we must adjust our attitudes to foreseeable situations so that we view them in a more realistic light. It is, you see, the *way* you look at things that arouses your feelings.

Take Janet, for example: 'I took one look at the long-haired lay-about my daughter brought home for tea and I was sickened with shock. How could she see anything in him? You know, typical student outfit, overcoat from Oxfam miles too big worn over faded jeans. Immediately I went onto the attack. I despised the lad before I'd even exchanged a few words with him. That night I couldn't eat my supper, and didn't sleep a wink. Couldn't touch my breakfast. Then my husband got mad at me. Told me not to be silly and invite him round to get to know him better. I'm glad now I did. And I should have more faith in my daughter's judgement. Now we all have great times together. He's really a nice chap, and so helpful to Dave in the garden'.

Is there anything we can learn from Janet's experience? Doesn't it show that, up to a point, our emotions are subject to our control? Those who have studied these matters say we can indeed change the way we feel about something by describing it differently to ourselves. They say there is no real need to react to people and places from first impressions and the way we interpret them. Obviously we must expect to have these emotional reactions but also we must be able to control them so that we can see things clearly and not coloured by biased opinion. In this way we are not as likely to get churned up inside.

Cultivating this attitude of mind, a cool, clear-headed objective approach might not be as easy for women as for men. Traditionally, it would seem women are always less likely to conceal their feelings: they do cry more readily, blush more frequently and collapse into giggles at times. And what a good thing too. Don't we all feel better after a good cry or giggle?

Somewhere between the dull, stiff-upper-lip person and the lively, emotional, easily-upset one, there is the ideal, healthier way to be. We can alter the course of our emotions, make them stronger or weaker, divert them into less dangerous channels. We can deliberately laugh, for example, at a rude remark or news that really angers us. Laughter can defuse a situation before it blows up into something worse.

So, gradually you can learn to separate personal feelings from problems so that they can be seen in a way that is logical and less likely to upset your emotional balance – and through this imbalance damage your health in more ways than one. With a serene mind and body at rest all systems will be at go for your rejuvenation. The next best thing you can do to ensure that the renewal process goes ahead smoothly is to see that you get the best from your sleep.

Getting the best from your sleep

Deep sleep is the great restorer, 'chief nourisher in life's feast', writes Shakespeare. And it is the most important healing agent of all. For centuries we have been led to believe that it smoothes away all lines of tension and has a benign effect on both body and mind. But the important thing to remember is that sleep comes in varying depths. You may appear to sleep all night but only for a part of that time – usually the first few hours – will you be in a deep sleep. This conclusion has been drawn from studies of brain wave patterns taken when subjects were asleep. Many doctors believe that many of the recuperative effects of sleep come from the time spent in the deep sleep stage. Some people, for example, can go to bed late, drop into a deep sleep right away and still get up fresher than the unfortunate ones who go to bed early and lie for hours without dropping into a deep sleep.

Of course, this makes nonsense of Benjamin Franklin's well-known jingle, 'Early to bed, early to rise, makes a man healthy, wealthy and wise'. And it perhaps explains why the amount of sleep needed varies so much from one individual to another. British Prime Minister Margaret Thatcher, for example, is reported to go to bed at 2am and get up again at 6am. However, the important point is to get to know how much sleep you personally need. And then you must have it in full or tell-tale signs will appear – irritability, impaired judgement, and muscular weariness.

On the other hand, it is possible to over-indulge in sleep merely as an escape from boredom. Ideally you should go to sleep when you feel tired and get up when you wake naturally refreshed.

Sometimes sleep evades those who are worried or under stress. They lie quite wakeful worrying about one problem after another until in desperation they get up for a drink or a walk around the house. The next morning they think that they are too tired to tackle the problems of another hectic day. They fear being unable to cope, their confidence breaks and they become casualties of stress.

There is no need for this to happen. The worst thing you can do is to get worried about not sleeping. If you miss a night's sleep you will make it up another night. Alternatively you can make it up with supplementary sleep.

Supplementary sleep

When you go to bed doesn't really matter. What does matter is that you get the ration of sleep you need every 24 hours. You can take it all at once or you can have it in separate sessions; some at night, some at midday and some in the early evening.

We need the oblivion of sleep to 're-charge' all our systems and eliminate the toxic products of fatigue. We do not necessarily need long hours of unbroken sleep which for some people seems to be an impossible luxury. If your sleep is habitually disturbed do not worry. Some doctors claim that broken sleep is often more refreshing than one long session.

How to improve the quality of your nightly sleep

The first obvious requirement is to invest in a good bed and pillow. Spend a long time in making your choice – not too soft and not too hard. Talk to people, try the bed in the shop.

A cold bedroom is not conducive to restful sleep, neither is a hot stuffy one. Many people find that a warm bath just before retiring to bed is helpful in relaxing the body. Try to get into the habit of a familiar routine; do not work until the last moment, potter about preparing yourself so that you are mentally unwinding. Resolve any problems before getting into bed or decide to push them firmly to one side until the morning. Have a good book by the bedside and fill your mind with this kind of trivia, driving out business and domestic problems. A light snack and warm drink before bed can be helpful.

Sleeping pills

Sometimes doctors prescribe these at times of extreme stress or to restore a natural rhythm into the sleep routine, but drug-induced sleep never seems to be quite as refreshing as natural sleep. Sleeping pills should not be relied upon as a permanent constituent of life.

Which is the most restful sleeping position?

Some lying positions place unnecessary burdens on muscles and can cause tensions, strain and pain. Lying in bed normally requires the minimum expenditure of energy because the pull of gravity on various parts of the body is counter-balanced by the support given by the mattress to nearly all segments of the body. If, however, the springs of the bed are soft and the mattress sags then the weak intervertebral muscles and ligaments have to work overtime. Eventually they become weaker still, stretch, and back-ache begins. In the treatment of almost every form of back-ache a firm bed, often with bed boards, is used.

Another important point about your sleeping posture is the position of the pillow. If you have two or three thick pillows arranged so that the head is placed in a position with neck muscles stretched then the tension induced in them prevents from resting. The advice given by specialists in this field of kinesiology is that the pillow should be of a thickness that keeps the head and neck in one line, with the pillow filling the gap between the tip of the shoulder and the neck. In sleeping on the side the pillow can be bunched and for sleeping on the back it can be flattened.

It is worth spending some time in finding out how you can get the best from the time you spend in bed – nearly a third of a lifetime – for relaxation and sleep can, coupled with the right attitude of mind, ensure that you are constantly renewing those parts of the body that suffer most from the wear and tear of everyday life.

To summarise

1) Your mind can work wonders for you. Have faith in its miraculous powers to revitalise your body.
2) Free yourself from emotional stress and give your body-powers the chance to work under ideal conditions – retreat and relax mentally and physically when you can.
3) Take time off for occasional breaks – midday, weekend, and for holidays. An essential part of the secret of self-renewal is knowing when to take a break – and taking it!

12   TAKE A BREAK

Journalist Katharine Whitehorn of *The Observer* recently wrote grumpily about the lack of sofas and couches in offices and ladies' rooms. A quick break in the middle of a terrible day can, she says, make all the difference between struggling on and packing up and going home.

Her column brought a quick response from the British Holistic Medical Association who agreed with her absolutely and told her how they ensured a quick break at midday. Regardless of the volume and the pressure of work, they take the 'phone off the hook, exercise briefly to release the tension in hunched shoulders and then lie flat on the floor in peace and quiet.

The floor can be surprisingly comfortable at midday especially if you can put something to act as a pillow in the hollow of your neck. Indeed, why not a pillow? You can feel muscle groups relaxing tension immediately. Let your legs fall lightly apart, arms away from your sides, palms of the hands falling upwards.

'Calm down, don't take your Valium®, stay in charge of your own health,' say these doctors of the BHMA, clearly practising what they preach. 'We are all convinced that this midday break has meant the difference between being able to cope with a non-stop day at full pressure and going under.' It's worth trying.

Can you manage a quiet nap in the middle of the day? Take a close look at your job. Is there a bolt hole where you could rest quietly for a short while? It would make a world of difference to your efficiency, your promotion prospects and, above all, your ability to stay young longer. Like one of the most famous British Prime Ministers for example: 'By some magic the man managed to retain the zest of a young man throughout a long life. Yet he broke all the rules – smoked interminably, drank, went to bed late, often working until two in the morning. Nevertheless it was as if there was in him some spring of ever-renewed vitality such as flows only in youth,' wrote that perceptive philosopher Professor Joad. The man? Winston Churchill.

Britain's great wartime leader was often described as a man with limitless energy. Where did all this phenomenal vitality come from? Joad did not tell us, but Eleanor Roosevelt gave the secret away. She described what happened whenever Churchill visited the White House during the most critical years of the war. *He took a break.* Every afternoon he took a long nap and woke up refreshed, full of vigour and ready for the hard work of the evening and much of the night.

Businessmen, actors and all who work late at night find that taking a break for sleep at some part of the day is a boon. It releases tensions, refreshes fatigued muscles and, which is perhaps most important of all, it helps to prevent the body from becoming over-tired. It is this that etches in your face the deep lines of weariness that are so ageing.

By taking a break the heart gets a chance to slow down its heart rate and the body can catch up with the debt of fatigue that has accumulated and eliminate it.

Once you begin to get some supplementary sleep you'll soon notice the difference in the way that you look and feel. There are times, though, when you will need a much longer break. A holiday.

Tranquillity works wonders

There is a moment at the start of a good holiday when all cares seem to slip away and everything takes on a slightly dreamlike quality. Is it really happening? Bags are stowed, you settle in your seat and for the next few days you begin to unwind.

It doesn't matter what you are doing: lazing on the sun-soaked beach turning like a sausage at allotted times, bargain-hunting in the bazaar or having an action-packed family holiday. The benefts come just the same. You are cut off from potentially harmful demands of other people and the pressure of work which have been battering at your defences for months. You have escaped to another world, even if it is only 50 miles down the road.

Now your body can get on with its marvellous recuperative work: renewing its energy and repairing tissues damaged by disease, overwork or physical inactivity. Tranquillity works wonders. So, within the short space of a few days' holiday you begin to look better and feel better. Holidays really are worthwhile.

But they are not only good for your health. You come back with new ideas – about the house, about work, about your future. It gives you time to think things through and you come home refreshed in body and mind alike. Holidays are a good investment.

Some people, however, get delusions of indispensability. It boosts their ego to 'hold the fort' whilst others take a break. 'It's all right for some, but I'm too busy to go away.' How wrong they are is not always evident until they are forced to stay away by sickness – often for months.

Everyone needs a rest from time to time. Your body warns you with symptoms of chronic fatigue, headaches, short-temperedness, irrational anger, digestive disorders, changes in heart rate and rhythm to name but a few.

If, after an especially difficult patch or tough period of work you feel shattered or exhausted then you've been given a hint to take things easier. Heed such hints. Your body is like a bank account. When you spend more energy than you've put in you overdraw your account. And you are in trouble. Your tiredness, whether physical, mental or emotional, is nature's way of warning you that you have reached the end of your endurance. Take a break!

Take two holidays

Many large industry groups now employ medical consultants to safeguard the interests of the firm by looking after the health of senior executives. It is sound commonsense to husband the experience and industrial leadership of successful directors. They are hard to replace. With this aim in view doctors frequently recommend top management personnel to take two holiday breaks a year. They need not be long ones.

Quick to appreciate the significance of this trend, travel firms push their persuasive advertisements through the colour supplements. 'When the air is sub zero and the outlook bleak it's a good time to take a second break. Cheer up those chilly days . . .' Often the advertisement is subtly aimed at the wife: 'How to spring-clean your husband' and 'a tired face is a frightening thing. If your husband has one take him away for a second holiday. After it he will work better, look handsomer, live longer.' Good business propaganda but sound commonsense too.

Planning a second holiday, even a long weekend can bring a warm glow into a dull winter's evening. It is worth the effort.

Planning and preparation

'We just packed our bags, dumped them in the car and set off south for the sun, without any route or plans at all. It was a wonderful holiday. Fourteen days at a little fishing village on the west coast, not even marked on the map. The food was fabulous, mainly fish of course, and ridiculously cheap. Miles of beach, beautiful sea and sunshine every day. When we came to pay the bill — what was it dear? I forget now, but we thought the old lady had made a mistake and only charged for one week . . .'

You've heard the story before? It is like the stock stories of 'my operation' which become more remarkable after each telling.

You *can* hit the jackpot and have a wonderful holiday by sheer good luck but it is safer and more fun to plan. Remember you are spending something more valuable than money — time. Sometimes it's not just your own but your family's as well. What might they all get from the holiday? Happiness, health, memories.

Only a rash or superhuman writer would claim to present a plan for a perfect holiday. There are so many variable factors — the weather, expense, food, other people. Personalities clashing can cause annoyance. Can you stand your friends for a fortnight? Think things through, plan and then prepare for what you are going to be doing whilst you are away.

Active holidays

There is little danger of physical strain from taking a more active holiday provided you don't leave your desk or car-seat one day and think you can climb a mountain peak the next. You need to prepare yourself.

If you intend to trek over fells, ski on alpine slopes, or swim under clear Mediterranean waters with a bottle of air strapped to your back, then get yourself in trim physically well beforehand. Then your enjoyment will not be marred by excessive stiffness or exhaustion in the first few days.

An active holiday project provides you with an ideal purpose for getting really fit and keeping fit. It will give an added zest for life. What better excuse for taking an evening off regularly each week to learn the techniques of some holiday sport. There are dry schools where novices can learn to bend, sway and use the skiing muscles. Large towns have sub-aqua clubs where you can practise snorkel and aqualung techniques in heated swimming pools during the winter months in preparation for the more exciting weekend and holiday expeditions in the summertime.

Not all active holidays demand physical preparation. Painting, photography, archaeological exploration, language study, pottery and glassware collecting, are examples of activities which can provide a motivating interest in the holiday plans which may eventually provide more pleasure and satisfaction all the year round. They can also be a healthy way of providing a counteracting force against the pressures of work.

Derek Manton found a more exciting solution to the pressure problem. He was a huge rollicking man of 38 with a full-lipped moustache, an ex-rugby player who had kept himself fit with squash and never had a day off work in his life. And then they reorganised the firm, 'rationalised' it for greater efficiency. Which meant redundancies for some and double the work for those who remained. That was bad enough. But when they knocked down his office walls and left him exposed, with all the traffic of paper and people from other departments howling around him, he knew it was time to take a break. In more ways than one.

His friend, Peter, an active union man, smiled knowingly and called it a management ploy, 'constructive dismissal'. And he gave a pithy piece of advice: 'Take time out, and think this thing through. It's all a matter of survival.'

Derek nodded thoughtfully. Recently he had been feeling distinctly seedy, not sleeping properly, never without a packet of indigestion tablets in his pocket and rarely free from nagging pain just beneath his right shoulder blade. No longer was he the robust, confident, youngish-seeming man he used to be. And although he was not particularly fond of alcohol there had been times lately when he felt like getting absolutely 'stoned', just for the devil of it.

So, for the first time in his life he descended to guile. He simply did not go into work the next day. He telephoned the office and left a message that he had an upset stomach . . . 'Must have eaten something that disagreed with me, or else I've picked up a sickness bug from somewhere.'

To forestall any subsequent questions he went to his doctor, one of the old school. And he talked. 'I'm a tolerant man, doctor, and I've learnt to take the bad with the good but even saints have their limits.

86

I've reached mine.' A thorough examination followed. 'Get dressed now,' said the doctor. 'I don't think you have anything really to worry about, I'll give you a prescription of Magnesium Trisilicate to settle your stomach, but what you really need is a break. You're under stress. Take the rest of the week off. And relax.'

When he got back into his car, Derek Manton felt for the first time in months a stirring of excitement, a rising feeling of exhilaration. Thoughts tumbled over themselves. Why not? He was a free agent, no longer married. Why shouldn't he take a real break? Not let the beggars grind him down. For 15 years he had let himself be tethered to his job in which holidays had been hurried interludes of gulped summertime between work and yet more work.

OK, that's it, he thought, and drove directly to a travel-agent. He booked a flight to Heraklion, Crete. He went home gleeful as a schoolboy, packed and dealt with outstanding domestic chores.

In the early evening, two days later, he was being greeted by a white-haired lady of the kind you read about in books, and being led into an old white-painted house with blue shutters, a bright, clean and not too expensive pension. Next door was a taverna and a few yards away the sea.

That night he slept tranquilly. In the morning he threw the curtains wide open and let the sunshine stream in. He glanced at his watch. Seven o'clock. The time immediately reminded him of his old routine; the alarm, the rushed breakfast, packed underground train, and the bustle of work that now seemed so senseless and far away.

'If there is one plane I have a right to miss in my life,' he thought, 'it's the one from Heraklion next week'.

All this was a long time ago. Derek Manton stayed in Crete. He misses his squash but he has many other equally enjoyable activities in the fresh air. He takes various little jobs in the summer that tide him over the winter months. He is happy and fit. He has indeed taken a real break. A possibility for us all to consider. We might not depart for exotic climes, but a complete short break away from our environment can work wonders. It could avoid some of the health hazards and emergencies that 70 per cent of us mid-lifers will have to face sooner or later. As we shall see in the next chapter.

To summarise

1) You're in charge. Blow the whistle when you've had enough.
2) Take time out for a 'psychological' breather.
3) There is more than one kind of break – investigate all possibilities.
4) This is your life-time. Plan it carefully.

13 QUICKLY FIT AFTER SURGERY

The letter had come unexpectedly. He knew it would come sometime but he was surprised it had arrived so soon.

Dear Mr. Grant,
Arrangements have been made for your admission and a bed reserved for you in Ward 15 on Monday 17 December at 10.00 am.
If you need assistance to get to the ward please report to the reception desk at the main entrance . . .

There followed further instructions. Enclosed was a blue booklet – 'Patient's Guide' which was 'to answer some of the questions you may have about your stay in hospital.' He had followed the instructions, packed his bag with essentials: pyjamas, dressing gown, slippers, towels, personal toiletries, disposable razors.

And so it was that shortly before ten o'clock on that bright December morning, Duncan Grant approached the glass doors of the District Hospital. They slid open automatically and he walked into the large carpeted hall. But he did not go to the reception desk. He knew the way to the ward and walked jauntily down the long corridor, not a bit worried about the date with the surgeon the next day. He had seen it all before. His friend had been in for exactly the same operation a month before. He knew there was nothing to it.

Leaving the lift he walked into Ward 15, pausing to let a nurse with a wheelchair pass. There was a relaxed atmosphere about the place. Morning medication had been given, rounds were over, some nurses had gone for coffee and others were quietly writing their case notes. A student nurse approached.

'Mr. Grant?'

'Yes.' His voice held a note of surprise that they really were expecting him.

'This is your bed. Get into your pyjamas and nurse will be along to see you.'

Efficiently and quietly the procedure commenced: the nurse took details of next of kin, telephone numbers, gave him an identity wrist band and hung a chart on his bed. A young white-coated houseman came next and checked him all over – heart, lungs, swollen ankles? Do you smoke? Any heart problems? Then he pulled out a broad felt pen and drew two large arrows down Grant's bare abdomen. Next came the Registrar, more checks, and finally the anaesthetist. Nothing was forgotten. And each time the wrist band was checked with the notes on the clip board.

'Right then, we'll be taking you to theatre early tomorrow morning. About 9.30 am.'

Preparations

75 per cent of the population need an operation at the start of mid-life. It helps to know something about what happens. The old saying is: 'Knowledge dispels a fear'.

Sometimes the operation will need to be done urgently and with little warning. At other times there will be time to prepare. An enjoyable and effective way of preparing yourself for an operation is to take a healthy holiday for a few days beforehand. Do not work right to the last moment if you can possibly avoid it. Allow some time to take a bit of physical exercise, gently, to improve your 'wind' and tone up the muscles without causing too much fatigue. Keep away from people with coughs and colds. If you catch a cold it could mean postponement of the operation.

A holiday will take your mind off the thought of what is to come so that mentally as well as physically you are as refreshed and fit as possible. It is your best way of co-operating with the surgeon.

Stop smoking if you can. Cut down on alcohol. The anaesthetist faces bigger problems with the heavy drinker than with the person who never touches alcohol or who drinks only in moderation. A period of abstinence from drinking alcohol before the operation can help to speed your recovery.

Smokers usually have a cough although many think they have not. When the habitual cough and bronchial tickle is accentuated by the irritation of the anaesthetic, the risk of rupturing abdominal and thoracic sutures is increased. Bouts of coughing can cause stitches to burst. If internal ones are affected then another operation might be necessary. Apart from the coughing hazards there are also the possibilities of respiratory complications such as pneumonia and bronchitis, to which the smoker is more prone.

Fat is a bugbear for the surgeon. If you have time and are overweight then go on a diet and lose as much as you need. It is overweight people who tend to develop post-operative complications.

Obviously, when an emergency operation is necessary there is no time for this physical preparation and therefore if you keep in trim all the time, you are likely to have fewer problems and a more rapid recovery.

Additional preparations

Before going into hospital 'clear your desk', think ahead, and make arrangements for what is likely to be needed at work and in the home. Make sure there are no domestic bills that are unpaid and likely to cause problems as a result. You don't want to come home and find your electricity cut off or court orders. Get someone else to take over the responsibility for a while. Very few people are absolutely indispensable. You will be back at work sooner if you have no worries whilst you are in hospital.

Also, and it is not being unduly pessimistic, make a will. This does not increase the odds against you or indicate a predisposition to leave this land for a better, but it would relieve your mind of a possible worry. It is something which should be regarded in the same way as taking out an insurance policy to protect your family. To die intestate throws an unnecessary burden on your dependants.

Getting better

When the operation is over you might need some physical rehabilitation with a physiotherapist or remedial gymnast. Gradually confidence will be restored with the development of physical strength and mobility. A visit to the physiotherapy department can prove to be a cheerful part of the day for patients. Little by little you will be able to take over your own rehabilitation programme. Get moving. Walk a little more every day. Breathe deeply. Plan your recovery programme so that you can get out into the fresh air during the best part of the day. Getting fit should be your first priority. Nothing else matters more than this.

You have to be firm with yourself. Think positively. Let nothing dampen your determination. Keep well away from the Jeremiahs in hospitals who take pleasure in filling you with morbid details of their own disasters. Stop their stories and walk away to dwell on brighter subjects.

The road back to total fitness is quicker for some than for others. It depends on so many factors – age, severity of the sickness and surgery, and basic constitution. Do not worry if you seem to be making slower progress than another. You are probably doing better than someone else.

The important thing is to be *fully* fit before going back to work. And here you will have to be resolute. In the final analysis it is up to the individual to decide when the right moment has come to go back to work, for rarely are there any half measures at work. When you're back, you're back and that's all there is to it. Don't be foolhardy and think you are doing somebody a good turn by going back to work before you are really fit enough, or you might find yourself back where you started.

Make the most of your period of recovery. It will give you time to think, read more widely, develop new interests. It is all part of the business of living and getting yourself physically and mentally fit enough to meet the challenges of life outside the hospital again.

Naturally, there will be times when a second operation may be necessary. But have faith – in your surgeon and yourself – no matter what your condition might be. People are always making marvellous recoveries. They do not give in, but win through even against the odds.

To summarise

1) Think ahead. Prepare yourself mentally and physically for the operation.
2) Keep away from people with coughs and colds before going into hospital.
3) Stop smoking, cut down on alcohol, and lose excess weight.
4) Clear your mind of worries before going into hospital.
5) Have faith. Think positively about recovery.
6) Be patient. Do not try to rush back to work too soon.
7) Rehabilitate yourself through progressive and gentle exercise as soon as your doctor permits.

14   WHY JOIN THE CORONARY CLUB?

The Berlin flight was delayed. Gordon Derby bought a newspaper, read the departure times again, and fumed. He wandered back between the counters of blonded girls lounging behind bottles of duty-free perfume. Now the ache in his chest was definitely there again. They had wined and dined him elegantly though not unwisely. Perhaps it was just indigestion . . .

He sat down, stretched his legs – deliberately not restricting the circulation by crossing them – loosened his tie and closed his eyes. The pain would now go, he was sure. It had done three weeks ago when he was at the sales conference. By the time Flight 427 to Berlin was announced he felt refreshed. No pain. Life could go on again as normal.

Three weeks later on a sales mission to Leeds, England, he felt unwell in the clothing factory, a queasy feeling and the ache in his chest again. His forehead was speckled with sweat, his breathing laboured and he wondered if he was going to faint. Within an hour, in a taxi on his way to the station, he was in severe pain. He called to the taxi driver. 'Hospital, quickly please.' A glance over his shoulder was all the driver needed. He knew where to go. 6 minutes later he turned off the main York road into the long tree-lined avenue that led to Killingbeck. An unfortunate name, he always thought, for one of the best heart hospitals in the country.

Seconds later he was being lifted gently onto a bed in the Coronary Care Unit. Contact discs were placed on his chest and wires looped from them onto a visual display unit where a white dot began to bounce across the screen as it registered his heartbeat. A doctor slid a needle into his wrist. On the end of the needle was a small plastic tap with a cap on the end. Through this, in an emergency, drugs could be fed directly into blood returning to the heart.

It was all done so smoothly, like watching a well-drilled squad in action. By night and day for almost a week that screen was under constant surveillance by medical staff. There were blood pressure checks, electro-cardiograph checks, blood samples taken for analysis, frequent examinations by the consultant and house doctor. All very reassuring. Everyone was willing to answer his questions.

Five weeks later Gordon Derby came out of hospital a different man. Thinner and wiser. In his hand he carried a yellow paper listing dos and don'ts. The most important taboo was smoking. 'If you're a smoker, STOP. If you're not, don't start.' Emphatic medical advice. And we shall see why.

Convalescence was leisurely. It had to be. And what surprised him most, perhaps, was that everything went on quite well without him. It left him wondering why on earth he had pushed himself so hard. Who cared? He was dispensable.

It was four months before he went back to work. But not to the old routine. The words of his doctor still rang in his ears: 'The guiding principle for recovered coronary patients is to be as wise as serpents and harmless as doves.' No longer did he curse or blow a gasket when planes were delayed and plans went wrong. He had developed a sensible respect for the other 'C', the big killer, coronary heart disease. He had learnt to guard his heart.

What can you do?

Gordon Derby had every reason to treat his illness with respect. He did not want a second heart attack. He knew that though most people have a deep-rooted fear of the 'Big C' – cancer – it is the other 'C' – cardiovascular disease – that is the biggest killer. The number of deaths every year from cardiovascular disease is more than twice that from all forms of cancer. 80 per cent of all deaths are due to it. Most of the victims are over 40. The message is clear. The longer you can stay 39 the better.

Those in Britain are at greater risk than other Europeans. The figures are frightening. For every Frenchman that dies of heart disease there are 10 Scots, or 10 Irish, or 8 English. Are you going to be one of them? There is no need. The Western European world would be well advised to take note of the way that death rates in the USA and Australia have fallen by about one quarter over the past decade. Changes in life style, particularly related to diet and smoking, have brought about this improvement.

You can guard your heart, protect and conserve it so that you can

94

lead a longer and healthier life. But you must act now. 'It is a sad human failing to leave things until they are too late,' says eminent heart specialist Dr Keith Bell, and adds, 'We take better care of our motor cars than we do of our heart'. But by some elementary precautions and the occasional checkup we can add years to its performance. We must avoid the well defined risks.

Do you know what happens when you have a heart attack? Think of your heart as a very strong muscle about the size of your clenched fist. It has been working, contracting and pumping, since you were in your mother's womb. For this it needs fuel – oxygen, and energy – food, brought in the blood through small arteries. These coronary arteries, as they are called, sometimes get narrower, 'furred up' like water pipes in a hard water area, by a disease known as arteriosclerosis. Now note, it is a disease and not just the natural process of growing old that does the damage. A disease we bring upon ourselves.

The artery wall thickens as fatty substances and cholesterol are deposited on it. Suddenly there is a blockage. Blood carrying life-giving oxygen cannot get through to the heart muscle. It stops contracting. Death comes without warning. Some are luckier. They survive, though the heart is damaged as muscle fibres deprived of oxygen die.

All this can be avoided. Or certainly it can be delayed until much later in life. How? By:
1) Stopping smoking.
2) Reducing body weight.
3) Changing your diet.
4) Exercising the heart muscle regularly.

Avoiding the risk factors

It can be argued that certain families are more prone to heart attacks than others, so that cynics say the best way to avoid a coronary is to choose your ancestors carefully. But what they fail to see is that it's not health characteristics we inherit that cause the trouble but *habits*. We grow up living like our parents live; eating similar meals, drinking, smoking, spending our leisure time as they do. We take the same risks.

If your family has a history of heart attacks then avoid the risk factors which are now well established and recognised by leading heart specialists. Let us look at these risks.

95

Cigarette smoking

In men over 45 smoking causes four out of every five deaths. With younger people statistics are even more convincing; there are more heart attacks among young smokers than among non-smokers of the same age.

When smoking became less popular in the USA in the early 1960s after the Surgeon General's report on the effects of smoking, there was a 20 per cent drop in the incidence of coronary heart disease. Findings of another research group in Framingham, Massachusetts, showed quite clearly that when fewer people smoked there were fewer heart attacks.

More factual evidence comes from blood tests. Cigarette smoking raises the level of certain compounds — lipoproteins — in the blood that are related to coronary artery hardening. From there it is a short step to heart disease.

Strange though it may seem these blood tests give new hope to those who decide to quit the smoking habit. Stopping smoking brings a reduction of lipoproteins in the blood which matches the figure it would have been if they had never smoked. Other independent tests also give hope to those who wonder whether or not it is too late to undo the damage of years of heavy smoking. *It is not too late.* Heavy smokers who have stopped for five years have almost the same chance of survival as those who have never smoked. Do not believe otherwise. It is worth stopping.

Journalist Stacey Brewer, who had survived a heart attack himself, will testify to this. A non-smoker himself, a fact which he believes saved his life, he was back in the general ward after four days in the Coronary Care Unit where he couldn't help hearing a succession of doctors and nurses warn another patient in the strongest possible terms that if he didn't stop smoking he would kill himself. 'A glance at the death list notices in the Evening Press a few weeks later proved they were right,' said Stacey later describing his experience.

You would think that the daily sight of white-faced patients — men and women — at death's door and of the less fortunate being wheeled through it, would put people off smoking for ever. Not so. Some still persist. I remember well, during a month of visiting a patient at Killingbeck heart hospital seeing dressing-gowned figures slithering off in their slippers to the loo for a sly drag in the afternoon and evening. Dicing with Death. And as we have heard, losing.

Diet

We are constantly bombarded with statistics which show that if we eat a lot of rich fatty foods we are more likely to have a heart attack. We are told that in countries where poverty keeps people poorly fed there are fewer heart attacks. But in the same countries — for example in China and Sri Lanka — higher up the social scale, where people are enjoying a better standard of living — there is an increase in the number of heart attacks.

Overweight, obese people certainly run greater risks. The golden rule must be to keep your body lean without becoming altogether a food faddist. At 39, you ladies are not subject to heart attacks as much as men. But what are you doing to protect the man in your life? Are you feeding him to death? Remember, being a widow is tough financially and emotionally; watch his diet carefully.

Whether we like it or not, we are all caught up in social systems such as family, work group, and neighbourhood. Everybody behaves more or less in response to the pressures and expectations of those around them. And, as a result, we are all subject to stress of some sort or other.

How we react to this stress affects the risk of having a heart attack. This aspect of stress is discussed fully in chapter 9 and all that needs to be said now is that we must be practical. It is very difficult to change your personality to reduce the risks associated with stress. No matter how much we say to ourselves that we must not get het up, must not get angry, must not shake the lemonade bottle so that it fizzes over — if we are made that way and a stressful situation arises then it probably happens.

The only sure way of avoiding this dangerous cycle of emotional upsets is to avoid those situations altogether. And this is not easy. It takes courage. For often it means giving up a job or a relationship, a difficult decision at any age. But in middle life it is very hard. Consequently it can be put off. Only you can make that decision.

But let us end this chapter on a more optimistic note: a message of hope from heart specialist Professor Shillingford. It should bring cheer to those who have already had a coronary — (and it happens to people in their 30s now more than it used to do). He says, 'It should be emphasised that if a patient survives the first few hours of a heart attack he will, in the majority of cases, make a complete and satisfactory recovery.'

As the older gangster film star, Edward G. Robinson, said after his second heart attack: 'You have a heart attack and it puts you to the side of the road for a while. Then you get up and go on.'

To summarise

1) Learn how to cope with stress.
2) Avoid a fatty diet.
3) Do not smoke.

Not asking a lot, is it? Chapter 16 will tell you how to stop smoking.

15 AVOIDING CANCER

The sound of the nurse's quick step receded down the corridor until it was lost in the silence of the Los Angeles hospital. The time was precisely 0135 hours on the morning of 12 June 1979 and the biggest ever box-office draw of the cinema had just died.

Displaying his true grit to the end, denying himself painkillers so he could say his last farewells to the family and friends, the tough, archetypal hero of 100 Westerns, John Wayne, took his final curtain call.

15 years earlier, in 1964, surgeons had cut half his cancerous left lung away and Wayne emerged from hospital with the headlined words: 'I have licked the big C!'

During the next 15 years he went on to direct films, act in them, and give active support to the Republican Party's presidential campaign for another film cowboy, Ronald Reagan. And it was also during this time that he had further operations to remove his gall bladder, to take part of his stomach away, and for a heart bypass.

In the course of his film career he had played soldier, aviator, adventurer and big-game hunter. And he had smoked 100 cigarettes a day.

When he had his final public appearance to collect the 'Oscar' for *True Grit*, and partly for the way he had − to use his own euphemism − licked the big 'C', he was so moved by the ovation that he almost broke down, saying: 'That's just about the only medicine a fellow every really needs.'

But there is a better medicine that avoids all the surgery and pain. It is called, 'Preventive Medicine', and it is the sure way to beat the big 'C'. You can take it. Now.

Beating the big 'C'

This year could be a crucial one in your life. Now could be the time you decide *not* to be one of the millions who die from cancer every year. Specialists tell us that three-quarters of all cancers are self-inflicted. We bring them upon ourselves. This year, now, you could decide not to be one of this afflicted group.

Case histories show that three out of every four cancer deaths are due to self-indulgence – physical and emotional. If we change our habits we can reduce the risk of contracting cancer dramatically.

This is the message being punched home by more and more cancer specialists. Will people listen to them, or take false reassurance from the free advice of friends who have only partial knowledge? It's anybody's guess. One cancer specialist, Dr Jan de Winter, with 30 years' experience of treating the disease, says that of all those who die from cancer 37 per cent do so from eating the wrong foods, 30 per cent from smoking, 7 per cent from sexual behaviour, and about 3 per cent from drinking excessive amounts of alcohol. There you have it: 77 per cent of all cancers which could have been avoided.

Much is now being done to help the recovery of those already afflicted. Convincing evidence of progress being made comes from all quarters. No longer need we fear the cancer diagnosis as the death knell it used to be. New drugs and methods of treatment now restore a high percentage of patients to a normal life. But the basic and most effective weapon in the fight against cancer is education, an increasing public awareness of the fact that cancers come from self-inflicted wounds.

For the servicemen in a wartime hospital the three capital letters: S.I.W. appeared on medical documents of those evacuated from battle zones due to their lack of care or deliberate wounding of themselves. This shameful S.I.W. stamp covered frostbite, during the battle of the Ardennes in 1944, and Venereal Disease during the Italian Campaign, as well as deliberately putting a bullet through a foot. 'S.I.W.' was, and still is, a Court Martial offence. How many of us would be found guilty of carelessly inflicting a serious injury upon ourselves? Today it is almost impossible to pick up a newspaper or magazine without reading an article about harmful habits which affect our health. We are aware of the risks but seem to live on cloud nine believing that cancer is something that only happens to other people. Suddenly it can happen to you.

It is a bad medicine to wait for diseases to happen. It is a recognised fact that for every patient found to have cancer there is another in the same locality about to discover a lump or significant symptom. What we must do is to take care now. Anticipatory care. And we must believe that we can avoid many of the cancers and the premature ageing that goes with them. Prevention is better than cure: it is more certain and less painful.

Over the past years we have been regaled with reports which show how bad our eating habits are. Our intake of fats and sugars is horrifyingly high compared with many countries in the east where there is a much lower incidence of cancer. Breast cancer mortality, for instance, goes more with the obese than with the slim. Excessive consumption of fats – particularly milk fats – is said to be responsible. Skim the milk and you cut the risk of both breast cancer and uterine cancer. Gone are the days when we can look upon the two inches of full cream on the top of a milk bottle with great pleasure in the belief that we are getting value for money. Give the cream to the cat and live longer yourself.

Skimmed milk has about half the Calories as full cream milk but identical nutritional value; in proteins and carbohydrates. Experiments with mice have shown that by cutting food intake altogether fewer cases of breast cancer develop. Similar trends can be seen in tribes in Africa who live on a meagre diet.

The other principal cancer found in women is cancer of the cervix. The key to reducing this risk seems to lie in the examination of statistics relating to which groups of women are likely to be afflicted. And there is no doubt that sexual behaviour is linked to cervical cancer. Prostitutes suffer most, whilst nuns and virgins seem to be spared. Advice given to women by cancer specialists is to use a barrier cream, keep to one partner who is meticulous about his hygiene, avoid sex during a period and have a thorough warm wash after intercourse.

Who is not aware now that the tar gases that come from smoking tobacco cause lung cancer? How many intelligent people still kid themselves that the relationship of smoking and lung cancer has yet to be proved? There is only one way to cut the risk of contracting lung cancer; stop smoking. It is not difficult. You will feel better and look younger. The way to drop this expensive and fatal habit once and for all time is described in chapter 16.

When heavy drinking is combined with heavy smoking there is a curious interaction which produces other cancers than those of the lung. They are found in the mouth, pharynx, larynx and oesophagus.

Signs of hope

The picture is not all grim. There are hopeful signs that people are forsaking life-threatening habits. More people are giving up smoking. Major retailers and supermarket chains are now putting pressure on manufacturers to produce healthier 'life-saving' foods. Retailers are realising that people are beginning to heed the startling evidence in the British government's diet report from NACNE[1] that the typical Western diet puts all of us at risk of getting various cancers, as well as heart disease.

What dietary action should we take? In a nutshell, as a population we should cut our fat intake by one quarter, sugar and salt intake by one half, and alcohol by one third. We should eat twice as much fibre and starch – that is, more cereals, wholemeal bread, more fruit and vegetables, especially jacket potatoes and leafy green vegetables.

Personal characteristics likely to cause cancer

Are certain types of people more at risk in contracting cancer? They are. This is the opinion of a large body of medical practitioners. Emotional upsets, such as bereavement, divorce, losing a job, moving house against one's wishes, are frequently linked with the onset of cancer, says Dr Jan de Winter.

But what can we do about these upset feelings? We can vent them. Dr Susan Blake, a psychiatric researcher at King's College Hospital, London, is reported as saying that, 'It is often said that people who bottle up their feelings are more cancer prone.' Right! We must give voice to these feelings. Get rid of them by talking them out.

This is the belief also of many doctors now practising the 'holistic' or 'whole person' approach to the treatment of cancer. It is based on the age-old concept that mind and body are inseparable and that we must harness the powers of self-healing which are within us all. To do this the doctor and patient need to explore the whole background to the disease.

'The main thing is for patients to realise that they are responsible for themselves and they should start to mobilise their inner resources and self-healing,' says Dr Alec Forbes, formerly consultant physician who

[1]National Advisory Committee on Nutrition Education, 1984.

set up the Cancer Help Centre in Bristol in 1980. Colleague, Penny Brohn, who suffered from breast cancer but recovered, said: 'Therapists feel that the very fact of having enough time to talk allows patients to unburden themselves of much of the anxiety that compounds ill-health and hinders recovery.'

What holds good for treatment is equally important for prevention. And what we are left with is this: in the fight against the big 'C' – cancer – there is a great deal we can do for ourselves. But we must act now with preventive medicine.

The body wants to be well and will be if we live in tune with it!

To summarise

Six ways to cut the risk of contracting cancer

1) Do not smoke. (More important than all the other factors.)
2) Drink no more than four units of alcohol daily (one unit equals a glass of sherry).
3) Avoid obesity. Eat more fibre, fruit and vegetables, and less fat.
4) Women should have a cervical smear every five years. (Or every three if sexually very active.)
5) Do not get acutely sunburnt.
6) Avoid emotional stress. Accept emotional situations if you cannot get away from them. But remember, he who fights and runs away lives to fight another day.

Observing the six factors of preventative medicine is not going to give you a permanent feeling of deprivation. Quite the opposite, in fact; you will be getting more out of life. In every way. Smoking is the one factor specialists say is the most dangerous of all the six factors, but it is now easier to stop. The sure way is described next.

16 STOP SMOKING

You can stop smoking if you want. Millions have done so. And they have added 10, 20, and even 30 years to their lives. This is not theory but fact. How is it done?

There are two stages. First you really must want to stop for good reasons. Secondly you must follow the method which specialists have proved to be successful. Ignore the free advice from friends who have failed themselves. Two thirds of all smokers have tried to stop at some time in their lives but less than half succeed. Now there is new hope. A new treatment.

But first let us look at stage one – being determined to stop for very good reasons. There are plenty of them and all convincing. They cover health, sex, money and social benefits.

Why stop smoking?

1. To live longer

You cannot bury your head in the sand any longer and say that the case against smoking as a health hazard has not been proved. Look again at the facts. Statistics are difficult to grasp especially when the talk is in terms of thousands, hundreds of thousands and millions. It does not make a tremendous impact to read that more British World War 2 soldiers have died and are dying from the effects of smoking than were killed by the combined armies of Germany and Japan. Nor does it shock you perhaps to know that among 1,000 men and women who smoke, six will be killed on the roads whilst 250 will be killed before their time through smoking.

But wait until you see Uncle Joe dying. Flesh fallen from his body leaving his limbs like broomsticks, unable to eat, unable to drink and having a dry parched tongue moistened with wet lint. And watch his pain-twisted face when he's in need of the next morphine pill. Then it makes an impact. The one personal case. It is unforgettable; I don't want to see anyone else suffering like that. Once is enough.

104

There's no point in fudging the facts. They have to be faced. And here is a nasty one. Of every four people who undergo an operation for lung cancer only one survives for as long as five years. Cigarette smoking kills 50,000 people a year in Britain. The death rate from lung cancer in Britain is twice as high as in the USA where a high proportion of the population has stopped smoking. But lung cancer is not the only health risk. Heart disease and bronchitis are also attributable to smoking cigarettes.

Death from chronic bronchitis is 20 times more likely amongst those smoking 25 cigarettes a day than among non-smokers. It is not only the smokers themselves who die either. Each year in Britain 1,000 babies die at birth or near birth because their mothers smoked whilst pregnant. Women who smoke whilst carrying a child are twice as likely to miscarry.

'Ah yes . . . enough . . . we know all about the figures . . . but my uncle smoked like a chimney and lived to be 93 . . .' And here the cynic will hunch his shoulders and wave his hands expressively Italian-style as if to say that figures don't count.

And so it is that intelligent, well-meaning folk will push away the horrific catalogue of painful deaths awaiting the persistent smoker. And reach for the reassurance of another cigarette. It only happens to other people anyway.

2. *To avoid sexual impotence*

According to a group of French doctors, a common cause of sexual impotence for men in their late 30s and early 40s is smoking and a diet high in fat. Both these factors affect circulation and, say the doctors, a poor circulation often results in failure to achieve an erection. Just as smoking causes narrowing of the heart arteries it also causes constriction of blood vessels in the penis. And a narrowing of the penis arteries by as little as 25 per cent is enough to prevent an erection.

This discovery can bring new hope to some men in despair, for this kind of impotence can be reversed by giving up smoking and changing to a fat free diet.

Naturally the French discovery will come as a blow to the cigarette firms who have for years promoted smoking as sexy and macho. It could also justify another warning on the cigarette packets and advertisements in addition to 'Smoking can damage your health' – *'Smoking can damage your sex life'.*

Research by the French medical team stressed that this kind of impotence was not just a problem for the middle-aged but also for the younger man not usually troubled in this way. Men in their late 20s.

Ironically, sexual impotence could prove to be a more motivating reason for stopping smoking than the risk of an early and painful death. But that's the way some people are made.

3. For tax relief

Why elect to pay more tax than you need? Think of the cash you are needlessly giving to the government every year. You could put aside that money and watch it grow and you could also use it to give yourself and family a bonus treat occasionally.

Your future will certainly look brighter financially in every way, the moment you stop. You'll be free from an expensive habit. Free from the worry of having to remember your cigarettes and matches whenever you go out. Free from the worry of wondering if there is going to be a shop open when you run out. And you'll be free from the worry that you may be killing yourself!

4. For your family's and friends' sake

You are a much nicer person to sit alongside when your clothes and hair don't smell of stale tobacco smoke. There is another point to consider too. Your non-smoking family and friends are not likely to relish the risk they are running from 'side-stream' smoking. For although the main risk is to the smoker, non-smokers who live with a smoker run a higher risk of getting chest disease.

The benefits for your family and friends begin on the day that you stop smoking and they go on for a lifetime. It is worth it. Remember the slogan: '*Kiss a non-smoker and taste the difference.*'

Positive signs

Recent surveys show that 80 per cent of smokers want to stop. You will have plenty of support.

Two out of every three who stop say they never miss smoking and that eventually it was easier to stop than they at first thought. Public opinion is now swinging against the smoker. Seats for the non-smoker are now more plentiful on public transport, cinemas, theatres and restaurants.

By now you should have reasons enough to stop. But how can we help people like Mike, a teacher, who wants to stop but can't? One day he said to me, 'I'm now 35, I watched my dad die at 66 from cancer of the lung. It was a horrible sight and you would have thought it would have cured me from smoking. Well it did. But only for a few months. I have two children and I want to be fit enough to play ball games with them and run about and grow old with them. I wish I could stop smoking but every time I seem to have kicked the habit someone offers me a cigarette at a staff meeting and I'm back where I started again.'

His story is typical of many. They know they are risking their health yet they keep on smoking. Why? It surely is not because of any of the psychological reasons given for younger people smoking – 'sophisticated thumb sucking', a feeling of inadequacy and the need to imitate the attractive glamorous celebrity or the 'he-man' portrayed in the tobacco companies' advertisements. The reason that mature people find difficulty stopping smoking is probably because they feel dependent upon some subtle ingredient in the cigarette smoke itself which they believe could be nicotine.

And this is where the really good news comes. If we could remove this feeling of dependency, this 'need' for the fix of the next cigarette, then stopping smoking could be easier. Well, that problem has now been solved. You can have your nicotine fix without lighting a cigarette. A new aid is on the market which can help you to stop smoking almost painlessly.

After 10 years of experience in most European countries a chewing gum containing nicotine has proved to be a risk-free aid to stop smoking. It is sold as 'Nicorette' and for some people in special need it can be obtained on the National Health Service. For most people though it can be obtained with a doctor's prescription from chemists.

As the gum is chewed a steady but small supply of nicotine is released and absorbed through the membrane of the mouth, thus satisfying the smoker's need without risk to the lungs. But it is no use thinking that Nicorette in itself is going to be the sure-fire cure. It is an *aid*. The first stage, remember, is motivation – the determination to stop smoking – and then comes the decision. Nicorette can make that decision easier to maintain.

The simplest and most effective decision to make is to stop completely. Cutting down is more difficult and a greater strain on the nerves, causing more irritation. You make only one decision: to stop –

once and for all. In any case, cutting down does not necessarily mean that you will be smoking much less for medical tests have shown that people who cut down the number of cigarettes smoked actually inhale more deeply and smoke them down to smaller stubs without thinking, in order to top up the nicotine level to what it used to be before cutting down.

It will help if you remember that smoking is a habit which is usually associated with certain times and places. If you break these links, you can break the habit more easily. Work out how you are going to cope with the danger spots, the times when cigarettes are going to be handed round. Be positive. You are a non-smoker. Plan new activities to replace smoking – things to compensate for the tingle of the smoke, things to do with the hands, and ways of coping with tension. Sometimes it helps to make an agreement to stop with a friend or relative. (Weight watchers find group motivation is a great help in slimming.)

Plan your 'D' day well – the day you are going to stop and make sure it will be a day when you are not likely to be under stress nor subject to the temptation of being offered cigarettes by others. On the day before you start, get rid of all your smoking kit – cigarettes, ash trays and lighters. You are not going to need them for yourself again.

Nothing succeeds like success. When you have spent one smokeless day you will know that you can do it. If you feel the urge to smoke, then immediately do something else. Distract your mind from the thought of smoking. Go to places in the evening where you would not think of smoking – the theatre, library, swimming pool. It is worth making a big effort during the first few days. Sooner than you think the craving will go away, particularly if you are using the Nicorette aid.

But don't ever think that you are cured for good and that you can allow yourself the occasional cigarette. You can't. It's all too easy to slip back to smoking as many as before.

To summarise
1) You can stop smoking if you want to stop. Think carefully about the effects on your health and sex life.
2) Reap the social benefits – people will like being near you better than when you smell of stale cigarette smoke.

3) Use Nicorette at first to get over nicotine dependency.
4) Stopping altogether is easier than cutting down.
5) Plan your campaign carefully and see it through. And remember, it's harder to say 'no' when you're out at night having a drink.

17 HOW ABOUT A DRINK?

'I'd been on the water wagon for a few months, but I still couldn't get rid of this terrible fear,' said Joanne. 'It was a kind of anxiety hanging over me that something terrible was about to happen. They said I'd get over it once I stopped drinking but months after my last drink I was still at the stage when a knock at the door, or the telephone ringing, would panic me into a cold sweat.

'My doctor sent me to a hospital which has a psychiatric unit where I had umpteen sessions with a "shrink" but even after that I still could not get rid of this ever-present fear, a kind of floating fear which had no explicable cause but got me dithering over even the simplest of decisions – like signing a cheque or making a telephone call.

'I never used to be like this. It started after being divorced and hitting the bottle, worrying that I was going into menopause and losing my looks. You see what puzzled me was that I had no real cause for this anxiety, no noticeable changes in my face or figure; I had money, a job, and a decent place to live.

'It didn't help when one of the doctors got angry and said I'd only myself to blame and I was being silly. Eventually, with the help of a more sympathetic psychiatrist from an organisation called "Accept", and with the support of fellow sufferers from "Alcoholics Anonymous", I was able to get back to a near-normal sort of life where I could make business calls on strangers without getting into a blue funk .

'But I don't kid myself that I'm cured. I know what the odds against that are.'

She was right. Recovery for alcoholics is not easy. We have all seen in the press the problems encountered by the famous: film stars such as Elizabeth Taylor, Richard Burton, Lisa Minelli, treated at the Betty Ford Clinic; international footballers like Jimmy Greaves and George Best; but we don't hear much about the tragedies of lesser mortals who wake up one morning and realise they are an alcoholic.

The symptoms vary. Joanne's problem was an ever-present anxiety.

Alcoholics often have irrational fears and anxieties that can make life a living hell. Fortunately for Joanne she recognised the signs early enough and got help. The symptoms could have been far worse. People who regularly drink five double gins, or five pints of beer, or its equivalent a day, run a risk of becoming seriously ill with, for example, heart disease, peptic ulcer, pneumonia, or cancer of the digestive tract.

Too much alcohol affects sexual potency – especially with men. As Shakespeare's porter said in *Macbeth*, 'Drink provokes the desire but takes away the performance.'

And remember, it's all too easy for the light-hearted, social drinker to slip into a pattern of heavy drinking. It is a short step then to becoming an alcoholic. You might never have been drunk. But you could still be an alcoholic. It could happen to anyone. It could happen to you!

Who is at risk?

Americans and Europeans alike are continually bombarded by ever more sophisticated advertising techniques. This means that the majority of us are frequently faced with a decision of how much to drink, whenever we go out socially to a pub, club, party, or friend's house.

And it seems that a lot of people are failing to make the right decision. As a nation, Britain is drinking more heavily. More and more alcohol is being produced. Brewers are investing millions in expanding plant and setting up chains of specialist outlets. The take-home trade is booming. Imaginative and persuasive advertising pushes up consumption and the brewers are laughing all the way to the bank, whilst booze-related diseases are increasing at an alarming rate.

The evidence is incontrovertible: whenever alcoholic drinks become more readily available, instances of alcohol-related problems increase. This was shown in Canada as early as the 1930s and 40s when the cost of alcohol fell by half and the death rate from cirrhosis doubled. A reduction in the legal age for drinking in the USA was followed by a dramatic increase in alcohol-related problems.

Over the last 10 years admissions to hospitals for alcoholic liver disease have gone up four-fold in some cities. A British Medical Journal report of April 1981 showed that offences for drunkenness and drink-driving have gone up frighteningly. Violent crimes, divorces and attempted suicides are all multiplying – and all these social ills have alcoholism as a major factor.

Why are people drinking more?

There are many reasons but the two main ones stand out more clearly above all others. Alcohol is cheaper now. It is easier to obtain. In relative terms – as a percentage of the average wage – beer and spirits are cheaper to buy than they were 20 years ago. A bottle of whisky worked out in this way is a third of the price it was then. Licensing restrictions have been relaxed. The number of off-licences has increased. Supermarkets are selling a wider range of drinks at temptingly cut prices.

Not surprisingly, women are suffering more now from alcoholism than was formerly the case. The bar is no longer a male preserve; more and more women go into bars and buy drinks openly. Moreover, because of the shift in employment opportunities it is often the woman of the household who finds herself shouldering the responsibility of being the 'bread winner'. She frequently finds herself managing not only a job but looking after a family. Perhaps predictably, a woman may turn to alcohol as a form of coping with stress.

More and more young people are seen to be at risk. One in twelve men or women between 35 and 45 is said to be drinking above the risk level, and where redundancies have thrown many people on the labour market there has been a distinct rise in alcohol-related problems affecting all age groups. Almost everyone is at risk.

So, how can we avoid being amongst the increasing number of people with a drink problem?

Guidelines for healthy drinking

1) Treat alcohol with respect; a little can give pleasure, a lot can bring trouble.
2) Try to eat something when you go out drinking. Even if you are not particularly hungry, nibbling a few nuts will slow down your rate of drinking.
3) Do not drink alone. If you go into a pub on your own, talk to someone if you can.

112

4) Avoid having another drink just because it's your round. Offer to buy others a drink or something else. Keep enough in your own glass to keep them company if you like.
5) Always dilute spirits well.
6) Choose a non-alcoholic drink sometimes. It often takes more courage to do this but why shouldn't you?
7) Set your own limits before you go out.

Remember that any fool can get drunk. It is not a sign of toughness or manhood or sophistication.

Alcoholics are not a race apart. They come from the ranks of ordinary folk who like a social drink, and then more, and more, and . . .

Help for the heavy drinker

People are sensitive about their drinking habits. Dire warnings are seldom heeded. We all know the feeling: It is far easier to give advice than to take it. Fortunately, though, there are ways of helping the heavy drinker to get back to a normal life where alcohol is no longer an all-pervading influence.

We have to accept the fact that the heavy drinker is usually well aware that alcohol abuse is changing his personality for the worse, harming his family and social life and ruining his health. But he still finds difficulty in doing anything positive about it. He accepts the situation as hopeless.

It is not. There is a road back. But you need to know the way. Doctors who specialise in helping people with a drink problem give the following advice.

To summarise

Guidelines for the heavy drinker
1) Aim for clear short-term goals that can be achieved without too much difficulty.
2) Take one day at a time. Do not think too far ahead.
3) Avoid emotional situations at home or at work which you know

have triggered off drinking bouts in the past. Work out new ways of dealing with them. Side step confrontations.

4) Try positive relaxation techniques to give you a feeling of tranquillity. Get into a routine of having a quiet hour.
5) Confide in your partner or friend and get help.
6) Enlist help from specialist organisations, such as Alcoholics Anonymous.
7) Above all do not be put off by an occasional lapse. It need not be catastrophic. It has happened to countless people who have eventually got back to a more normal life.

You're in charge

Eventually the heavy drinkers will reach the stage when they have to decide whether modified drinking is a more acceptable and feasible goal than total abstinence. Most specialists, though, favour a period without any alcohol at all until evidence of physical harm has disappeared.

Get all the support you can. Fill your time with other activities and note how much better you begin to feel once on the water wagon. It's your life.

18   BACK CHAT

On a bitterly cold, wet evening on the sea front of a Dutch fishing village, eight of the world's strongest men waited, kicking their heels whilst competition officials struggled to lift cases of heavy metal into the back of a red hatchback car. At last the door was lowered. 'Ready. Number One!'

Britain's Geoff Capes, the title holder, strode forward, pushed his wet hair back from his forehead, wiped his hands and then paused for a moment as if looking for a place to grip the long steel bar attached to the car's rear end. He settled his body ready, back straight, feet firm and a little apart.

Suddenly he lowered his body by bending his knees but at the same time keeping his chin tucked in and back straight. He grasped the bar. His legs straightened. The car rose on its springs, there was a loud blowing out of breath for the final heave and the wheels were clear of the ground. 'Good lift.'

One after the other they came as more weight was added. All massive men, each with his own distinctive personality. But all with the same stance. Exactly. Back straight, breathing freely and using the powerful leg muscles to lift the tremendous weight.

Now, you may not wish to enter for the 'Strongest Woman or Man in the World Competition' or anything like it but you could learn how to lift properly so that you avoid a good deal of needless suffering through careless lifting and carrying in the home. A tug, a heave, a snatch can tear a few muscle fibres or ligaments and so make you unfit for work or play. Another casualty for the back pain clinic. In pain, you move awkwardly, a classic picture of old age.

'How's your back today?' could be a question you'll soon be asking for there is not one street in the western world that does not have its martyr to backache, says a leading specialist. In fact back symptoms account for more visits to the doctor than any other problem.

Back pain, without warning, afflicts young and old alike. It is a universal woe that takes the spring out of your step and wipes the smile off your face. And you certainly look older than 39 as you heave yourself awkwardly out of your car seat after a long drive and tentatively try to straighten up without being suddenly pole-axed with pain.

Back pain can be sudden and excruciating or it can be a constant nagging that leaves your nerves shredded and your features lined. And it is no consolation to know that four out of five people suffer from it at some time during their lifetime. In a variety of simple ways it can begin; from stretching over to lift a heavy bag of groceries to picking up a baby's rattle. And you are caught, bent double with pain, unable to straighten up.

The causes of back pain

Your spine is a graceful S curve composed of a series of bones stretching from your skull to your tail, joined together by muscles and ligaments and separated from each other by small cartilage discs, which give flexibility and lubrication. Down a central canal in these bones, runs the spinal cord, a collection of nervous tissue which comes out between the vertebrae to various parts of the body. If any of these small bones or the cartilages separating them become damaged or displaced then the nerves in the immediate vicinity can become involved and cause pain or tingling sensations in the parts of the body they supply. Similarly, strain on the muscles and ligaments supporting the vertebrae also causes pain.

Apart from disc displacement, rheumatism – either in the muscles or spinal joints – is the main cause of backache. In acute or sudden attacks, the muscles of the back go into a protective spasm around the affected area to form a kind of splint which prevents further movement. They can remain painfully contracted for days. In severe cases bed rest is essential and a doctor should determine the degree of injury.

Sometimes the small muscles linking the separate segments of the spine and consequently the soft cartilaginous disc, which acts as a cushion between the bones, may bulge forward causing painful pressure on the sciatic nerve serving the lumbar region, buttocks and back of the leg.

For men and women who have to sit for long periods at a desk or wedged between the wheel of a car, backache is an occupational hazard. When your body is habitually bent forward the muscles between the vertebrae get stretched and they tear more easily when excessive strain is put on them. Lifting and pulling when the back is bent or stretched forward can suddenly catch you with a stabbing pain that indicates damage has been done. For example, the mother who leans forward and stretches over the pram handle to lift out a baby is putting herself in a typical situation for straining her back. Better to step round to the side of the pram.

Other causes of backache are kidney complaints, in which the pain may also travel down towards the groin, malformation of the spinal curve, and inflammation of the bowel.

Women have an additional cause for backache. During pregnancy and childbirth the strong ligamentous joints at the lower end of the spine and in the pubis relax in order to allow some movement and expansion. After the birth the stability of these joints is usually restored but there is sometimes a residual weakness. This means that the muscles of the back have to work harder to maintain stability and they eventually become painfully fatigued.

There is yet another cause of backache which was mentioned at the end of an earlier chapter – stress. Many doctors believe that a considerable number of back pain problems stem from emotional upsets. When emotions are suppressed they believe that muscles and blood vessels are constricted enough to cause pain in itself, often in the back, and that when the tension is relaxed the pain can vanish as suddenly as it began.

Prevention

Prevention is always better than cure. Avoid the causes, physical and mental, if you can. Keep your back and abdominal muscles strong through regular exercise. Try to adapt the working surfaces at home and in the office so that the spine is not continually bent forward.

If you have to spend many hours driving, avoid 'chauffeur's back' by using a clip-on chair back or put a pillow behind you to give firm support to your spine if your car seat is too soft. On long trips stop occasionally to stretch your legs and back and relax the posture muscles. Never sit for long in a chair with your back slumped in a curve. Doctors recommend back sufferers to stand up and walk about every 20 minutes.

People who have to sit and write for long hours at a time could adopt the American University method. Sit alongside the table or desk with the paper at your right-hand side (or left if you are left-handed) and in this way you can write comfortably whilst your back is supported by the chair back.

If you are overweight trim down if you can to what you weighed at 25. Extra poundage around the waist puts an extra pressure on the ligaments and muscles of your back.

Above all, learn how to lift and carry without putting too much strain on your back muscles.

Safe ways to lift, carry and push

Unlike the arm of a crane, the spine is not designed to carry heavy loads when it is in a horizontal position. It works most efficiently and with minimal danger of damage when it is held upright and straight by the postural muscles. The weight of the body, and any load carried, can then be transmitted directly through the vertebrae segments and cartilaginous shock-absorbing discs to the suporting pelvis and legs. (See Fig. 8.)

If you try to lift heavy weights with your back bent then you cannot make efficient use of the powerful leg extensor muscles in the thigh — as the strong men were doing in lifting the car. And if the leg muscles are working hard then the main effort is thrown upon the smaller muscles of the spine. Sometimes these muscles holding the segments of the spine together are not equal to the task and injury results.

Fig. 8   Lifting and carrying a heavy box

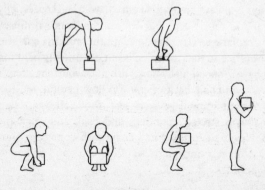

A typical situation in which such injuries occur is when you decide to tackle a neglected corner of the garden. You dig, tug and struggle with weeds and roots until suddenly a searing pain shoots out from the small of your back and takes your breath away. It is like being gripped by a giant whose thumbs are breaking your spine. You might be able to straighten up and stand but you will probably drop to your hands and knees, unable to move in a mounting spasm of pain the like of which you have never known before.

You can save yourself a lot of effort and minimise the dangers in lifting, carrying and pushing if you learn the techniques recommended by specialists who have studied the mechanics of muscle action in work study. Posters and instructional teams who visit factories have explained with success the safe and easy way to lift and carry awkward loads, and we can all benefit from the skills developed.

The fundamental principles to follow are:

1) Keep the back as straight and upright as possible.
2) Use the powerful leg extensor muscles.
3) Put your feet close to the object and about 12 inches apart.
4) Make maximum use of momentum once the object is moving but do not snatch.
5) Keep the combined centre of gravity of your body and the load directly over your feet.
6) Breathe freely throughout the movement.

Once your have had back strain you must take particular care of your back because torn muscles and ligaments are repaired with less resilient scar tissue than the original, which is liable to tear again.

Getting relief

The good news is that most backaches go away in a few days but it is nevertheless advisable to see your doctor if in doubt, for only he can advise on the right course of treatment, after considering the history of the trouble and making a physical examination. Early treatment can save months of needless suffering and worry. Sometimes quick relief can be provided by relaxant drugs.

Sleep on a firm mattress that supports the spine throughout.

Sagging beds can cause backache. Put a board between the mattress and the spring base, and see if that helps. It often does.

Bed rest is the best thing that you can have when pain is bad but take care how you lie. Flat on your back with pillows under your knees helps your spinal muscles relax. Otherwise lie on your side in the foetal position, knees up. If you still wake up with backache then put blankets on the floor to make a mattress and sleep on this for a few days. If the pain then goes away it might indicate that you need a new and firmer mattress on the bed.

Heat from an electric pad and aspirin can help to relieve the pain. Deep heat treatment in a hospital physiotherapy department can soothe the tender area and in chronic cases massage can be beneficial.

A boon for backache sufferers is the reclining chair. It is an ideal resting position, for the spinal muscles need not work to support the weight of the trunk and head, tension is taken off the hip flexor muscles attached to the spine and thigh bone, and all the muscles which normally have to work to maintain posture can relax. This relaxation naturally helps to relieve painful muscle spasm in the injured region of the spine.

It is not unusual for some people to find that nothing seems to bring relief. Do not despair. The Back Pain Association which has branches throughout England is always ready to help fellow sufferers and can advise on alternative treatment. (Headquarters: 133 Park Road, Teddington, Middlesex TW11 0AB.)

What is the alternative?

Back in the 50s and 60s, people who practised non-medical healing methods had labels attached to them like 'quack' and 'unorthodox' but now a truly remarkable change has taken place. The term 'Alternative' has been given more recognition by the medical profession. It is a name which covers methods which ally themselves to what has become known as 'Holistic' medicine. The Alternative treatment takes the whole person into account – diet, life-style, personal relationships, habits, emotions, posture. And all these important facets of a person are investigated before treatment is prescribed. Then, manipulative techniques may be used and adjustments to diet and life-style recommended. Other healing methods such as herbal, homoeopathic or acupuncture could be suggested too.

It is certainly worthwhile making enquiries about the alternatives to avoid the misery of recurring backache. Remarkable successes have been recorded when alternative treatments have been employed in the treatment of painful backs. But there is a proviso.

See your own doctor first to be sure there isn't a more serious problem that might otherwise be missed. He will probably be able to advise you where to go for alternative medicine – and who to avoid. There are some practitioners who advise you to keep paying them regular visits – and fees.

Rehabilitation

When all the pain has gone, and not before, patients in medical rehabilitation centres are often given exercises to do which help to prevent a recurrence of back pain. They are exercises to strengthen the muscles of the back and those of the abdomen which balance them. The exercises will also help you to feel more confident about your general fitness as well as your back. Try them. But always work within pain-free limits.

1) Lie face downwards with hands clasped behind your back. Lift head and shoulders off the ground. When you feel strong enough lift your legs as well.
2) Lie on your back with knees raised. Press elbows hard on the floor and arch your back as high as possible.
3) Lie on your back with knees raised and reach gently forward to touch your knees.
4) Lie on your back with knees raised. Bring one knee to your chest, lower to resting position.

When your doctor is sure that your back has made a full recovery he might advise swimming, cycling, and fast walking which are all easy on the back and improve general muscle tone. Always listen to your body – it will tell you through pain, either immediately or the next day, if the exercise has been too severe. This is perhaps the most important lesson to be learnt about the problem of pain: learn how to live with it so that it does not trouble you. Without being obsessively aware of your back do make a mental note about anything which seems to affect it adversely. And if there is a persistent symptom that troubles you then do not hesitate to go back to see your doctor in case there is a condition that requires more urgent investigation. Pain is often a way nature has of warning you that something is wrong.

Quick action can be essential for the cure of some of the more serious complaints; the old adage is still true – 'A stitch in time saves nine'.

To summarise

1) Seek your doctor's advice and give a detailed history of the pain as soon as it troubles you.
2) Remember most back pain disappears with rest.
3) Women have to be particularly careful before and after childbirth .
4) Beware of soft mattresses and chairs which do not give adequate support.
5) Strengthen your back with exercise when you are pain-free.
6) Avoid injuring your back in the first place by learning the proper way to lift and carry.

19   IT'S YOUR CHOICE

In the here today, gone tomorrow world of fad diet and fad exercise books, it's all too easy to become confused, and even cynical. Never before have there been so many books by people famous in other fields than health and fitness. Never before have there been so many contradictory theories and gimmicks of the 'eat as much as you like' or 'eat fat and grow thin' variety, etc., etc.

Fortunately these 'best sellers' have been balanced by a steady stream of convincing down-to-earth, reliable reports put out by the medical press: by the World Health Organisation and the American and British Medical Association, and the like, who are not out for a 'quick buck'.

Their energetic health education campaigns to keep the public well-informed are now bearing fruit. So that in the year that America's oldest president faced a fight for re-election at the age of 73 a truth dawned on the public at large. You can stay fit and active until much later in life − if you make the effort. And no longer need you fear being thought a hypochondriac for simply taking care of your health.

But it is not only the elderly who have suddenly woken up to this fact. The young mid-lifers are now beginning to indulge in the greatest health boom in history. They have caught on to the idea of life-prolongation through running, jogging, biking, and cutting cigarettes, caffeine and cholesterol. They are the converted. In their minds there is no shadow of doubt left that we are what we are because of what we have done, or not done, to ourselves. And they are absolutely right.

In the final analysis you are responsible for the rate at which you age. It is a variable rate determined by you. Age does not necessarily go hand in hand with decay. You *can* stay young longer. *It is your choice!* As Cary Grant once explained to a reporter who asked how he managed to retain his lissom sparkling youth in later life: 'It's just that other people persist in making themselves old with liquor, cigarettes and the wrong food,' − all a matter of choice.

There is a lot we can do ourselves. But we all tend to overlook the obvious and we need reminding at times that the human body with all its powers of endurance and its life-preserving capacities needs to work with some sort of assistance from us. Otherwise all the creams, lotions, dyes and powders in the world will not ward off the day when you look in the mirror and notice the tell-tale touches of time, the silent reminders that you are not as young as you used to be. Then soon comes the even sharper reminders – the breathlessness, loss of figure and all the aches and pains of the prematurely aged.

So, let your aim be clear: it is for 20 more years of youth, not an extension of decrepit old age. And for this you need to make decisions on how you are going to live. Firm decisions. Now. You cannot be fatalistic and leave it all to chance. Life is not a gamble, not a roll on a fruit machine drum. Life is a challenge. It must be met by positive action which can ward off the ageing process.

After 39, the years bring more responsibilities and you have to be physically and mentally fit enough to withstand the emotional stress they bring. Your capacity to cope with all this depends upon mental attitude and environment as well as physical considerations. Diet is not enough. Neither is exercise alone. What is needed is a comprehensive programme of everything that makes you feel happy and full of wellbeing. In fact it could be said that to be happy and content is half the battle. A cheerful outlook reflecting good health is the most important step, since looking and feeling younger is as near as you ever will get to actually being younger.

'You've got to work at staying young,' said Ginetta Spanier, Directrice of one of the world's most famous fashion houses, Pierre Balmain. 'It's not the number of years that counts, it is holding yourself straight. And not letting yourself go – especially fat. A sprightly walk helps. Not dragging your feet. Hopping up to fetch things, bending down to pick them up instead of sitting there with your arm out-stretched. Most important of all is zest for life.'

Now is your aim clear? It should be to bring your body back to its full potential of vitality and virility. You have the keys in your own hand to open the door to many more years of youth after 39.

What do you have to do?
Cut out smoking and heavy drinking and concentrate on the following three key areas:

1) Reduce your body fat to 15 per cent of body weight. How do you know what 15 per cent is? The pinch test will guide you. If you can squeeze out more than an inch of flesh from that hollow between the hip bones and ribs, you're too fat. Try also pinching the back of your upper arm between shoulder and elbow. Again, a fold of more than an inch means you are running a health risk.

   Being overweight causes problems from the relatively trivial to the fatal. From tiredness and aching feet to high blood pressure and heart disease. Taking off a stone or two can change your life in many exciting ways. Remember the equation: Calories taken in, minus Calories burnt in exercise equals Calories stored in fat. Whether you balance the equation or not, is your choice.

2) Get into exercise. Your body moulds itself to the life it leads. Without exercise joints lose their range of movement, muscles waste and your posture slumps. With physical degeneration there is often a psychological depression. You just don't feel like tackling problems if you are drained of energy and listless. Don't forget either the old axiom: 'Use it or lose it.' It is a law of nature: 'that which works, develops, that which does not, wastes.'

   You have read what the specialists have said about exercise. But they do not give you the most convincing argument of all. You cannot read it or hear it: you feel it. The exhilaration of feeling on top of the world. Trim and fit.

   Take three short exercise sessions a week and make sure your pulse rate goes up to about 100 or 120 a minute, whichever can be done without undue discomfort. For your heart's sake.

   Today, in Britain, 1 in every 10 men and 1 in every 19 women now aged 39 will die of a heart attack before the age of 65. America and Australia have got the message; there, the incidence of heart disease has been declining since the early 1970s. In Britain it is still the same. The British must work at it.

3) Learn how to cope with the gritty, abrasive effects of emotional stress. Life without any stress, of course, would be dull, but too much of it makes you a very different person, pallid, run down and weighed down by the cares of work and family responsibilities. In such a state you are not just likely to feel older and less fit but you actually will be biologically older.

   Running alongside Stress there is often his stable-mate, Depression. You begin to have doubts about your capabilities, become forgetful at work, and hesitant. And you begin to feel you have missed your chance in life. Get rid of that idea.

There is much you can do in the years before you. Women, like wine, mature with age. They are often more interesting to men after 39. And the same can be said for men. Broaden your range of interests. Mixing with younger people can help. And take your birthdays in your stride. They are useful as a day for taking stock in your life; for thinking about what you have done and where you are going. Break new ground. Get enthusiastic for a new venture if you can. It will prevent the years from catching up with you too soon.

Leading a full life certainly helps. In her 40s Helena Rubenstein built up a beauty business and at 90 wrote in her memoirs: 'Work has been my beauty treatment. It keeps wrinkles out of the mind and the spirit. It helps to keep a woman young.' Katie Boyle, television personality and magazine agony aunt agrees. At 58 she deals with 2,000 letters a week, is up to her neck in radio and television work yet still has that healthy, clear-eyed beauty that age just bounces off. She says: 'I've lived so fully that I never think about getting older.'

At 42, ballerina Margot Fonteyn formed a new dancing partnership with Rudolf Nureyev; Henry Ford was 50 when he went in for mass production on the assembly line. In art, we all know about Grandma Moses who only started painting at 78 and went on to make a million from her primitive rural scenes. But let us not forget Michelangelo who was appointed Chief Architect at St. Peter's Rome when 71 and went on painting his frescoes until he was 89. And there are Titian, Picasso, Matisse, Rouault, Braque, and Dufy, all of whom worked until their late years, forever innovating.

Sophia Loren, one of the world's most beautiful women, came to her 50th birthday with a feeling of surprise. Rich and famous, she need never work again, but that is not what she has in mind at all. She wants new roles, fresh challenges. 'My ambition,' she says, 'is to keep alive the same drive that has allowed me to achieve most of the goals of my life. At my age I still expect bigger opportunities than the ones I've had.'

Work can keep us young. But work can also kill. Today more and more people in their 20s, 30s and 40s are realising the real cost of getting to the top in this highly competitive world. 'The cost of anything is the amount of what I call life, which is required to be exchanged for it immediately or in the long run,' was how Dale Carnegie once put it. Or to put it another way, we are fools to pay more for a thing in terms of what it takes out of our lives and our health than it is really worth.

Some people can get all wrapped up in a job and are convinced that their work is the most interesting thing in the world. Fair enough. It will be good for them. But others seem to be driven on without heeding the cost. For them, work is not a labour of love but a worrisome ordeal, day after day as ambition pushes them onwards towards the celestial city called 'Success' without allowing them time to ponder the question: 'Is it worthwhile?' They risk ulcers, mental breakdown, heart failure. Yet the goad of ambition urges them on, often to disaster.

So, we are faced with the dilemma that work can keep us young and yet that it can kill us. What are we to do?

We must pause. At 39 we have reached the halfway stage of life. The years ahead are precious. It would be a pity to waste them. There is only one thing we can do. Take a long look at all the possibilities. Strip off the blinkers and look at what we might be missing. And if we find that work is becoming a health hazard decide it is time to put a sign on the door: 'GONE FISHING'.

It's all a matter of choice: yours! In the years ahead whether you stay young or not will depend on what you decide. It will mean balancing work with play, activity with relaxation, exercise with rest, and stress with serenity. And it will mean using all the other suggestions for health and happiness that have been emphasised in this book.

This is your life: play it your way. It is no dress rehearsal. One day, when you reach a great age, the oft-repeated question might be put to you: 'What would you do if you had it all to do again?' What will you say then? Will you be echoing Colette's words: 'What a wonderful life I've had! I only wish I'd realised it sooner.' Or maybe the ironic wit of Eubie Blake, the ragtime pianist who, on his 100th birthday said: 'If I'd known I was going to live this long I'd have taken better care of myself.'

It's up to you. Good Luck!

APPENDIX I: CIRCUIT TRAINING SCHEDULES

Full instructions on how to use these training schedules to obtain maximum benefit are given on pages 52 to 55. Study them carefully and remember that no matter how fit you used to be, it is probably a long time since you were in regular training. Don't be tempted to start with the more difficult exercises.

How to begin

1) Warm up with the six exercise routine shown on page 53.
2) Try the exercises in the first schedule until you get the knack of them.
3) Test yourself on each exercise in turn, to see how many repetitions you can do.
4) Take a breather between each test.
5) Record your score on the circuit training card – 'maximum repetitions' column.
6) Insert half your maximum score in the 'training task' column.

Start training the next day, but play safe and:

1) Never strain to complete an exercise
2) Follow closely the recommended rate of progress
3) Try to make training a regular habit – three times a week.

Schedule One

1) Head and shoulder raising: Lie on your back with feet a little apart, arms by the side. Raise your head and shoulders off the ground just as high as necessary for you to see your ankles. Lower down to the floor again. (Fig. 9(a)).
2) Trunk-raising backwards: Lie on your front with hands clasped behind the back and arms straight. Raise the head and shoulders as far from the floor as possible. Pull your shoulder blades together. (Fig. 9(b)).
3) Half knee-bending: Stand in front of a chair as though you were about to sit down. Bend your knees until your buttocks touch the seat and then stand again. Do not rest your body weight on the chair at all during the complete set of repetitions. (Fig. 9(c)).

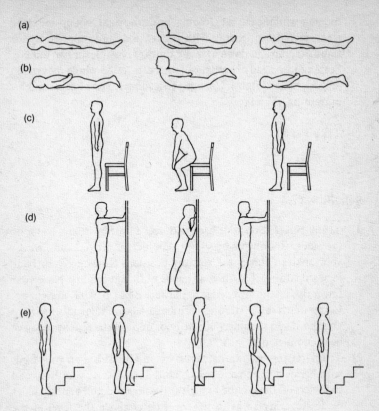

Fig. 9　(a) Head and shoulder raising
　　　　 (b) Trunk-raising backwards
　　　　 (c) Half knee-bending
　　　　 (d) Press-away
　　　　 (e) Stair-stepping

4) Press-away: Stand facing a wall, a little further than arm's reach. Lean forward to put your hands flat against the wall beneath the shoulders. Press yourself away until your body is clear of the wall and feet flat again, hands away from the wall. Fall forward into the starting position again. Do as many repetitions as you can before the exertion becomes too severe. Count the repetitions and make out the schedule according to the circuit training instructions. (Fig. 9(d)).

5) Stair-stepping: *Either* walk up and down the stairs in your house as many times as possible *or* stand facing the bottom stair. Step on to

the stair with the left foot leading, bring the right foot up and stand erect, step down leading with the left foot and followed by the right. Step up and down as many times as possible for two minutes keeping to a steady rhythm of four beats to the whole movement (left, right, left, right). Change the leading leg on alternate nights of training. (Fig. 9(c)).

Take it easy!

Schedule Two

1) Trunk-curl: Lie on your back with feet a little apart and hands by the sides. Raise your head and shoulders until you can just see your ankles. This is the starting position. Now curl your body forward and reach with your hands until you can just place your finger tips on the lower edge of the knee cap. Do NOT sit right up. Lower down to the starting position, as above. Remember to keep your head and shoulders off the floor until all the repetitions have been completed. (Fig. 10(a)).
2) Trunk-raising backwards, hands behind head: Lie on your front with hands behind your head, palms down. Raise your head and shoulders off the ground as high as possible and pull your shoulder blades together so as to lift the elbows above the level of the shoulders. Lower down to the floor. (Fig. 10(b)).
3) Knee-bending: Stand with arms by the sides and heels firmly on the floor, feet a little way apart. Lower down to a deeper full knee bend position as shown in fig. 10(c). Stand up. Do NOT lift the heels.
4) High press-away: Stand with feet well back from a heavy table or window sill, arms straight and supporting the body as shown in fig. 10(d). Bend your arms until your chin is just above the edge of the table and then straighten them again. The higher the table or support the easier the exercise becomes.
5) Box-stepping: Stand facing a box approximately 15 inches high. Step on and off as described in the stepping exercise of Schedule One. Do the exercise for two minutes. (Fig. 10(e)), or carry on with stair climbing increasing the number of completed ascents.

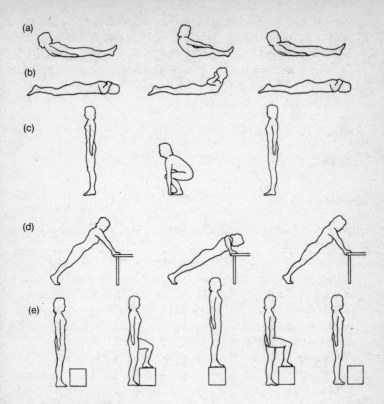

Fig. 10 (a) Trunk-curl
(b) Trunk-raising backwards, hands behind head
(c) Knee-bending
(d) High press-away
(e) Box-stepping

Schedule Three

1) Trunk-curl, feet raised: Lie on your back with feet supported on the seat of a chair or stool. Raise the head and shoulders off the ground and from this starting position curl forward to touch the knee caps with finger tips. (Fig. 11(a)).

2) Trunk and arms raising backwards: Lie on your front with arms stretched sideways, palms down or holding a small weight. (A tin of meat or milk will do initially.) Lift the head and shoulders as far off the floor as possible, at the same time pulling the arms backwards in line with the shoulders as shown in fig. 11(b).

131

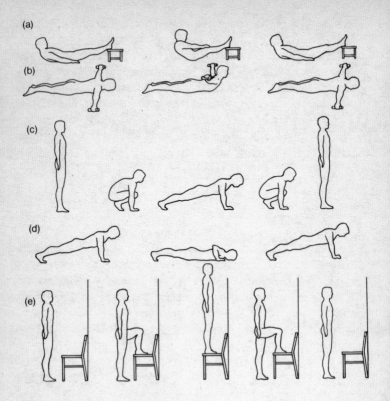

Fig. 11 (a) Trunk-curl, feet raised
(b) Trunk and arms raising backwards
(c) Burpee
(d) Horizontal press-away
(e) Chair-stepping against a wall

3) Burpee: This is a four movement exercise. From standing go down to the crouch position with the knees fully bent, jump the legs backwards until the legs and trunk are in line, then jump forwards to the crouch again, and stand up. (Fig. 11(c)).

4) Horizontal press-away: support the body by the hands and toes as shown in Fig. 11(d). Keep the body in one straight line with the legs, and the hands directly below the shoulders, fingers pointing forwards. Bend the arms until the nose touches the floor, and press up until the arms are straight again. Keep the body off the floor throughout the repetitions. Do not struggle when one arm appears

132

to be weaker than the other or wriggle upwards for an extra repetition.

5) Chair-stepping: Stand facing a chair which is stood against a wall. Step on and off at the rate of 30 times a minute for 2 minutes. Be sure to stand properly on the chair each time and keep to the rhythm left right, left right, for the duration of the exercise. Do not struggle to complete 2 minutes. Stop when you've had enough. (Fig. 11(e)). *Or* carry on with stair climbing, increasing the number of ascents.

APPENDIX II: 7-DAY SLIMMING MENUS

Now that we're all turning away from traditional fare to avoid the formidable list of diseases related to it, we have a golden opportunity for trying out new and exciting dishes which are both healthy and good to eat. Variety is the spice of life so now is the time to bring new ideas and new flavours into your diet. You can then look upon your slimming programme as fun.

Don't be put off. Experiment. Combine foods that you think might go well together. Many of the world's recipes came from accident or experiment. Get away from the old recipes – they were killing us anyway – and make up your own bearing in mind the basic principles that we know all about. Low in fat and sugar, high in fibre and with plenty of fresh fruit and veg.

Spice up your food. Garnish it attractively. What a difference there is, for example, between the simple boiled cabbage and that stir-fried in a little oil with onions and caraway seeds. Try out the new ideas you see in the magazines. Put into practice the basic principles of healthy eating to make meals that will keep you healthy and trim whilst being tasty to eat.

Right. Here we go. This dieting business is going to be enjoyable – like your exercise – or you'll never stick to it. To get off to a good start you can build your own diet menus around the seven main meals described below. Use the suggestions for breakfast and midday snack to complement the main meal of the day. When you have it is up to you. The emphasis is on flexibility. Do it your way!

Main Meals − **(all quantitites are to serve 4)**

1) Chicken Risotto

You need: about 12 oz/350g of cooked chicken
2 medium sized onions
1½ pints (850ml) of chicken stock (or use two cubes and water)
2 garlic cloves
2 tablespoons (40ml) of diced frozen peppers or 1 fresh green pepper, thinly sliced
5 fluid oz/150ml of cider or wine
3 oz/75g seedless raisins
4 oz/100g mushrooms
2 oz/50g walnuts
9 oz/250g long grain brown rice
black pepper
a little salt or lemon juice.

Remove any skin, scrape away any fat lying beneath it, cut the chicken into slices or cubes. Fry the onion until tender but not brown, add to the pan the peppers, mushrooms, walnuts and rice. Stir for about 3 minutes. Pour in the wine and boil briskly for a few minutes stirring all the time. Now add the stock, a very little salt, pepper, and stir well again before covering and allowing to simmer gently until all the liquid has been absorbed by the rice. It should then be reasonably fluffy and tender. Now add the chicken pieces and cook thoroughly. This is important. Do not just warm them through. 10 minutes will be needed. Serve on hot plates with fresh parsley to garnish.

Green salad and wholemeal bread go very well with this dish.

2) Baked Haddock Potatoes

You need: 8 oz/225g smoked haddock
4 large evenly shaped potatoes for baking
1 medium onion
1½ oz/40g margarine
2 oz/50ml yoghurt (Greek sheep's milk yoghurt is particularly good for this)
½ oz/12ml coarse ground mustard
2 oz/50g grated cheese
fresh parsley to garnish.

Set oven Gas Mark 6/200°C/400°F.

Wash and dry the potatoes. Prick several times with a fork to stop the skins bursting in the oven, lightly fry the chopped onion in vegetable oil or margarine. When the potatoes are baked (about 1¾ hours) cut into halves and scoop out the flesh into a large bowl. Stir in the fried onions and fish pieces, mustard, and yoghurt so that the mixture has a creamy but firm consistency. Heap the mixture into the potato cases, piling it up like a generous helping of ice cream in a cornet and return to the hot oven for 10 minutes. Remove, sprinkle with paprika and garnish with chopped chives. Eat the potato jackets which are rich in fibre.

3) Seafood Pasta Salad

You need: 8 oz/225g cooked prawns
10 oz/275g wholemeal pasta shells
1 tbsp/12ml vegetable oil
1 tbsp/12ml wine vinegar
black pepper, salt, lemon juice
1 tbsp/12ml grated lemon rind
2 tbsp/25ml chopped gherkins
2 tbsp/25ml sweetcorn
3 sticks of celery, thinly sliced
½ a red pepper thinly sliced
5 oz/150ml plain yoghurt
2 oz/50ml black olives
chopped chives to garnish.

Boil the pasta shells until just cooked (tender but not soft) – this will take about 12 minutes. Drain thoroughly and mix with oil, lemon juice and wine vinegar, salt and pepper. Mix together the sweetcorn, gherkins, celery and lemon rind. Pour the yoghurt over this mixture and stir gently into the pasta. Serve the seafood salad garnished with black olives and parsley.

Eat with hot wholemeal rolls, crisped in the oven or under the grill.
Follow with fresh fruit in season.

4) Red Kidney Bean and Vegetable Stew

You need: one 14 oz/400g can of cooked red kidney beans
2 medium sized onions
4 celery sticks
3 carrots

1 red or green pepper (or diced mixture of frozen peppers)
2 garlic cloves
1 oz/25ml tomato purée
one can 14 oz/400g tomatoes
5 oz/150ml beer or red wine
black pepper and a little salt
2 oz/50g margarine
mixed herbs, (basil, oregano, parsley are best)
Parmesan cheese

Prepare the carrots, celery, onion and pepper, slicing all thinly. Chop the garlic finely and fry all together with a little margarine. Add the beans, purée and tomatoes, beer or wine. Simmer gently for about 10 minutes or until vegetables are tender. Sprinkle grated Parmesan cheese on top and serve hot, with wholemeal bread rolls.

Follow with fresh fruit salad.

5) Tuna Nicoise

You need: one crispy lettuce
1 small tin of anchovies
One 4 oz/100g tin of tuna in brine
1 hard boiled egg
4 small tomatoes
1 small red pepper
black pepper
2 oz/50g French beans cooked
8 black olives
a few capers
a little finely chopped garlic
3 tablespoons of French dressing.

Slice the tomatoes into circles, cut the anchovies lengthwise, quarter the egg and divide the tuna into flakes. Slice the red pepper finely, mix the tuna, pepper, tomatoes, beans, olives, capers, garlic and black pepper with the dressing and arrange on the lettuce leaves in a salad bowl. Garnish with the egg and anchovies. Serve with baked jacket potatoes – or cold potato salad.

6) Beef and Haricot Casserole

You need: 6 oz/175g haricot beans soaked and cooked for 1 hour

8 oz/225g shin beef
2 medium sized onions
one 14 oz/400g can of tomatoes
1 clove garlic
1 teaspoonful/5ml paprika
2 teaspoonfuls/10ml wholemeal flour
half pint/275ml stock – (water plus cube)
lemon juice
2 tablespoons/15ml tomato purée.

Cut the beef into small cubes and fry in vegetable oil until brown, next fry the sliced onion and finely chopped garlic and cook until soft. Stir in the paprika and tomato purée, add the flour and stock and bring to the boil. Add the beef, haricot beans, lemon juice, and can of tomatoes. Bring it all to the boil again, cover with well fitting lid, and cook in the oven for 2 hours at 170°C/325°F, Gas Mark 3. You should then find you have a thick and tasty stew that is not too fattening.

Follow with unsweetened pineapple or fruit salad.

7) Spiced Liver Casserole
You need: 1½lb/700g calves' or lambs' liver
2 lb/900g potatoes
2 large onions
1 clove garlic
6 juniper berries
1½pt/850ml stock
¼ pint/150ml yoghurt.

Heat the oven to 200°C/400°F/Gas Mark 6.

Slice the liver, scrub and slice the potatoes, slice the onions, chop garlic finely, crush the juniper berries. Mix garlic and juniper into the stock.

Layer the liver, onions and potatoes in a casserole pan. Pour in the spiced stock. Bring to the boil on top of the stove. Cover the pan and cook in the oven for 1¼ hours. Stir in the yoghurt just before serving.

7 Breakfast Suggestions
1) French Omelette (to serve 4)

You need: 6 eggs
pinch of salt and pepper
½ oz/15g margarine
(for 'fines herbes' add 1 large teaspoon (5ml) of chopped herbs to the mixture).

Break the 6 eggs into a basin, beat with a fork until the whites and yolks are well mixed, add seasoning and a tablespoon (20ml) of water. Heat the pan well, drop in ½ oz/15g margarine, and, when frothing, pour in the eggs. Stir round slowly with a fork giving the pan a shake as the egg mixture begins to set. Lift the edges gently with a fork and when brown underneath, fold in half.

For a slightly more substantial breakfast omelette, add fried tomatoes seasoned with basil before folding over.

2) Muesli

To the plain oats add chopped walnuts, sesame seeds, sunflower seeds, raisins, bran and chopped dried apricot. Natural yoghurt can be added or milk to moisten.

3) Half a grapefruit

With one or two slices of wholemeal bread.

4) Porridge Oats

Cook with water and serve with skimmed milk. Do not smother with sugar. Add pre-soaked prunes or other dried fruit to give sweeter taste.

5) Fruit Salad

Chopped apple, orange, sunflower and sesame seeds. Followed by toasted wholemeal bread.

6) Grilled Kipper

A good start to the day. Full of vitamins and nourishment so have this on a day when the main meal is not going to be substantial.

7) Something Different

Why not try a bowl of hot tomato soup with a thickening of barley? You can add bran to this too, if you wish.

Ring the changes. Experiment with non-fattening healthy foods. Use skimmed milk in tea or coffee but also try some of the tasty mixed fruit teas now on the market. They need no milk or sweetener, and are very refreshing.

Suggestions for midday snacks

Packed lunches

These can be in salad form that can be forked from a plastic container. Combinations of chopped celery, apple, pineapple and cabbage make a tasty Florida Salad. You can add carrot, cucumber, beetroot, raisins, orange segments, cashew nuts, walnuts and turn it into more of a crunchy salad. Once you start experimenting there is no reason for being bored with your healthy midday salad. Rice and cooked beans can make it a little more substantial if you wish. Make your own dressings of oil and vinegar, yoghurt and a little mustard and lemon.

At home

You can cook if you wish: French onion soup with mixed green salad, baked potato with grilled cheese topping, tuna fish toasted sandwiches, bean and lentil soup with salad, spinach and poached egg, stir fry mixed vegetables with plenty of green leafy ones which are so good for you and good for filling without fattening.

Eat fresh fruit afterwards, especially oranges and apples for their roughage as well as vitamin content.

All these suggestions for a 7-day slimming menu give flexibility that allows you to have some control over your own diet. There is a wide choice of foods in many mouth-watering combinations so that dieting is no longer a chore. You will enjoy your mealtimes; soon you will get into the habit of eating healthy, satisfying meals that will keep you in shape. Choose the diet that suits your life-style, reduce the portions, and then you can whittle away the pounds without any apparent effort at all. You'll be a good loser! *And a winner as well.*

APPENDIX III: THE FIBRE CHART

Until recently fibre was thought to be an unimportant aspect of nutrition but in recent years research has shown it to be an essential part of a healthy diet. Here are some of the foods readily available and rich in fibre, graded on a 3-star rating.

Fibre Chart

Cereal Foods		*Vegetables*		
Bran	★★★	Beans: Butter	★★★	
Wholemeal bread	★★	Haricot	★★★	
Oat bran	★	Kidney	★★★	
Wholemeal pastas	★	Soya	★★★	
Semolina wholemeal	★	Black Eye	★★★	
Wholemeal soya flour	★	Baked	★★	
Breakfast cereals	★	Broccoli	★	
		Cabbage	★★	
Fruit		Cauliflower	★★	
Apricots, dried	★★★	Chick peas	★★★	
Figs, dried	★★★	Garden peas	★★★	
Prunes	★★★	Lentils	★★	
Sultanas	★★	Spinach	★★	
		Sweetcorn	★	
Nuts				
Almonds	★★	*Seeds*		
Coconut, dessicated	★★★	Sesame	★★	
Hazelnuts	★★	Sunflower	★★	
Peanuts	★★			

APPENDIX IV: PRESSURE LEVELS OF WORK

Rating is from 10 to zero: the higher the rate the greater the pressure.

Pressure Levels of Work

Miner	8.3	Farmer	4.8
Policeman	7.7	Armed forces personnel	4.7
Construction worker	7.5	Vet	4.5
Journalist	7.5	Civil servant	4.4
Pilot (civil)	7.5	Accountant	4.3
Prison officer	7.5	Engineer	4.3
Advertising personnel	7.3	Estate agent	4.3
Dentist	7.3	Hairdresser	4.3
Actor	7.2	Local govt. officer	4.3
Politician	7.0	Secretary	4.3
Doctor	6.6	Solicitor	4.3
Taxman	6.8	Artist, designer	4.2
Film producer	6.5	Architect	4.0
Nurse, midwife	6.5	Chiropodist	4.0
Fireman	6.3	Optician	4.0
Musician	6.3	Planner	4.0
Teacher	6.2	Postman	4.0
Personnel	6.0	Statistician	4.0
Social worker	6.0	Lab. technician	3.8
Manager (commerce)	5.8	Banker	3.7
Marketing/export		Computing personnel	3.7
personnel	5.8	Occupational therapist	3.7
Press officer	5.8	Linguist	3.7
Pro. footballer	5.8	Beauty therapist	3.5
Salesman, shop		Vicar	3.5
assistant	5.7	Astronomer	3.4
Stockbroker	5.5	Nursery nurse	3.3
Bus driver	5.4	Museum worker	2.8
Psychologist	5.2	Librarian	2.0
Publishing personnel	5.0		
Diplomat	4.8		

Chart produced by Manchester University Institute of Science and Technology, February 1985.

APPENDIX V: IDEAL WEIGHT CHART

Ideal Height/Weight

		Men			Women		
Height		Small Frame	Medium Frame	Large Frame	Small Frame	Medium Frame	Large Frame
ft	in	st lb	st lb	st lb	st lb	st lb	st lb
4	8	–	–	–	6 11	7 3	7 13
4	9	–	–	–	6 13	7 6	8 2
4	10	–	–	–	7 1	7 9	8 5
4	11	–	–	–	7 5	7 12	8 8
5	0	–	–	–	7 8	8 1	8 11
5	1	8 5	8 11	9 7	7 11	8 4	9 0
5	2	8 7	9 1	9 10	8 0	8 7	9 3
5	3	8 10	9 4	10 0	8 3	8 11	9 7
5	4	8 13	9 7	10 2	8 6	9 1	9 11
5	5	9 2	9 10	10 7	8 10	9 5	10 1
5	6	9 6	10 0	10 12	9 0	9 9	10 5
5	7	9 11	10 4	11 2	9 4	9 13	10 9
5	8	10 0	10 9	11 7	9 9	10 3	10 13
5	9	10 5	10 13	11 10	9 13	10 7	11 3
5	10	10 9	11 3	12 1	10 3	10 11	11 8
5	11	10 13	11 8	12 6	10 7	11 1	11 12
6	0	11 3	11 12	12 10	10 11	11 5	12 2
6	1	11 7	12 3	13 1	–	–	–
6	2	11 11	12 8	13 6	–	–	–
6	3	12 1	12 13	13 11	–	–	–
6	4	12 5	13 4	14 2	–	–	–

All weights include light clothing but no shoes.

Wrist measurements as a guide to frame size:

	Women	Men
Small frame	up to 6in.	up to 6½in.
Medium frame	up to 6½in.	up to 7in.
Large frame	over 6½in.	over 7in.

Statistics from insurance companies have shown that the death rate can rise by as much as 13% for every 10% a person is over their recommended weight.

INDEX

Abdomen, muscles of the 33-38
Alcohol 110-114
Ateriosclerosis 95

Back pain 34, 115-122
   alternative treatments for 120, 121
   exercises for 121
   prevention of 117, 118
   relief from 119, 120

Calorie requirements 25
Cancer 99-103
   causes of 99-101
   personality and 102
Cardiovascular disease 93-98
   diet and 97
   smoking and 96
Cholesterol 14
Circuit training 51-55, 128-133
Cycling 45-47

Dancing 49, 50
Diet 12-31
   menus 133-139
   slimming 25-29
   well balanced 15, 16
Drinking, heavy 113

Emotions, control of 77-79
Exercise programme selection 40-42
Exercises 35, 37, 38, 52, 53, 128-133
   enjoyment of 39-43
   rating 46
   time for 52
   warming up 53

Fatness, causes of 22, 23
Fatty foods 16
Fibre 17, 140

Garlic 14

Heart attacks 93-98
Holidays 82-88
   active 85-87
   planning for 85

Impotence 58, 105, 106

Jogging 11, 42

Lifting 118, 119

Nicotine chewing gum 107

Paunch, the 33-37
Posture 34
Pressure levels of work 141
Psychosomatic illness 64

Relaxation 70-75
   techniques 71-74
Relaxed lying positions 71, 72

Salt 17
Sex 56-61
Sleep 79-81
   position for 81
   quality of 80, 81
Sleeping pills 80, 81
Slimming 21-31
   exercise and 29
Smoking, stopping 104-109
Spine, the 34, 116, 117
Squash 47
Stair climbing 44, 45
Stomach flattening 32-38
Stress 62-69
   causes of 63-65
   relieving 65-68
Sugar 17
Surgery 90-92
   preparation for 90, 91
   recovery from 91, 92
Swimming 47, 48

Tennis 47
Tranquillisers 66

Ulcers 65

Vegetarianism 13, 20
Vitamins 18

Walking 48, 49
Weight, ideal 23, 142